P9-DWS-496

CALGARY PUBLIC LIBRARY

JUN -   2012

MENU CONFIDENTIAL

MENU CONFIDENTIAL

Conquer the Calories, Sodium and Fat
Hiding in the Foods You Love

MEGAN OGILVIE

Photography by Christopher Campbell

Collins

Menu Confidential
Text copyright © 2012 by Megan Ogilvie.
All photographs copyright © 2012 by Christopher Campbell, except where otherwise specified.
All rights reserved.

Published by Collins, an imprint of HarperCollins Publishers Ltd

First edition

The information in this book is intended for reference only and not as a substitute for dietary advice from
a knowledgeable health professional. Product availability and nutritional information is described as of the
time of writing; menus and recipes are naturally subject to change. Nutritional information contained in this
book has in most cases been provided by the restaurant; in other cases it is the result of testing a sample from
the restaurant by an independent lab.

No part of this book may be used or reproduced in any manner whatsoever
without the prior written permission of the publisher, except in the case of
brief quotations embodied in reviews.

HarperCollins books may be purchased for educational, business,
or sales promotional use through our Special Markets Department.

HarperCollins Publishers Ltd
2 Bloor Street East, 20th Floor
Toronto, Ontario, Canada
M4W 1A8

www.harpercollins.ca

Library and Archives Canada Cataloguing in Publication
information is available upon request

ISBN 978-1-44340-726-7

Printed and bound in Canada
TC 9 8 7 6 5 4 3 2 1

CONTENTS

Introduction

This is a book for every Canadian who eats away from home. That's all of us. For many, dining out is a treat. For others, eating a takeout sandwich is the only way to fit food into a busy schedule. But whether we're digging into a creamy pile of linguine alfredo or downing a chicken wrap at our desks, more and more of us want to know what we're putting in our bellies.

It's hard to make smart choices, though, when we don't know how many calories and how much fat and sodium lurk in our favourite dishes. Many restaurants do post nutrition information for their meals. But those numbers are not always easy to find—or to understand. (How much is 1,200 mg of sodium, anyway?) Some other establishments don't provide nutrition numbers at all, which leaves us wondering how many calories are hidden in an innocent-looking plate of spaghetti.

This is where *Menu Confidential* comes in. In this book you will find nutrition information for popular fare, from hamburgers and pizza to steaks and salads—and just about every food in between. You will also find out how many calories get crammed into a bag of movie popcorn, how much fat is in a convenience store snack and how much sodium has soaked into a pound of sauced-up chicken wings. When an eatery's owner has chosen not to reveal its nutrition numbers, I have sent the featured food to an accredited laboratory to uncover its calorie, fat, carbohydrate, protein and sodium content. Within these pages, you'll find information you can't get anywhere else.

For each of the more than 100 foods included in the book, I've translated its nutrition information and shown how, with easy tweaks or simple swaps, the food (or a similar choice) can fit into your daily diet.

Don't worry. The idea isn't to make you feel guilty about indulging in the occasional double cheeseburger or regret falling for that fresh-baked muffin you picked up with your morning coffee. Rather, it is to arm you with the information you need to choose more wisely from a menu and to help you easily navigate your local food court.

Sadly (for those of us who don't need to eat like Olympic athletes), almost every food we eat outside our homes will be two to eight times larger than a recommended portion size. That means many additional calories and much more fat and salt. And sometimes the lighter-looking choice—that chicken-topped salad, say—may be the most calorific on the menu. We've all been fooled many times.

The good news is that you can quickly learn to spot those hidden diet disasters. The even better news is that there are simple things you can do to make just about any food easier on your waistline. *Menu Confidential* will show you how to do both.

I know you will have fun gathering tips and learning new strategies. Flip through a few pages and you will find facts that will make you chuckle, maybe even shriek. (Would you guess that a platter of nachos has as much fat as 40 strips of bacon?) I also know this is the book you will turn to again and again, either for a quick reference check on fast-food french fries or for inspiration to overcome a particular dining dilemma. And I guarantee that by the end of this book, you will have learned to become a smart diner. Making better, more informed choices every time you dine out is the best defence against incremental weight gain.

The great thing about this approach is that there are rarely big sacrifices. Instead, the strategy is to make small changes each time you order, like swapping cream for milk in your coffee or ditching the bland processed cheese from your sandwich. Over time, these small calorie savings add up. This strategy also allows you to indulge without guilt. Splurging on an 800 calorie entree is okay when you've scouted out the nutrition numbers and adjusted the rest of your meal—and your day—to make it fit.

Become a smart diner and you will find it easier and easier to prevent extra pounds from creeping up and settling on your hips and around your belly. I promise.

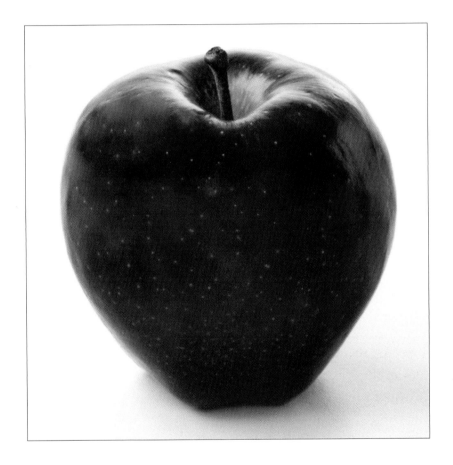

NUTRITION
101

None of us need to think about glycogen or lipoprotein when we line up for a sandwich. But some basic nutrition knowledge is key to figuring out which meal at a restaurant will best fit into our daily diets. In this short chapter, you will learn why your body needs calories, fat and other macronutrients, why consuming too much of them isn't good, and the amounts health experts say we need to aim for every day for optimum health.

It's a quick crash course, not a chapter out of a nutrition textbook. So it won't be tedious going. But if you are a nutrition whiz, you may want to skim the next few pages. Or if you want to find out right away how much fat is packed into movie popcorn, feel free to skip ahead. Just come back to "Nutrition 101," your reference guide, every time you have a question about your daily calorie needs or about why you shouldn't consume 3,000 mg of sodium every day.

>

Why our bodies need calories

What is a calorie?

In technical speak, a calorie is defined as the amount of heat required to raise the temperature of a litre of water from 14.5 to 15.5 degrees Celsius. No one other than a lab technician would think of a calorie that way. All we really need to know is that a calorie is a measure of the amount of energy derived from food.

Why does my body need calories?

Our bodies need energy to make everything inside us work. We need calories to power our hearts and lungs, to grow new cells and to monitor and adjust hormone levels—as well as to fuel hundreds of other basic body functions. About 60 to 75% of the calories we burn every day are used to keep these systems running smoothly.

Eating, among other things, burns calories. About 10% of our daily calories are used to digest, absorb, transport and store food. (Don't get too excited. This fact is not carte blanche to dig into a carton of dulce de leche ice cream.)

Moving, from playing a vigorous game of tennis to brushing our teeth, is the third main way our bodies burn calories. This is the greatest variable and the main reason why an Olympic cyclist needs to eat 8,000 calories a day—6,000 more than what the average office-going citizen requires.

What does my body do with calories?

The three main sources of calories are carbohydrates, protein and fat.

Our bodies digest these macronutrients differently, but each has the potential to turn into fat if the body doesn't need it right away for energy.

Very simply, our bodies convert much of what we eat—whether a baked potato or a bowl of chili—into glucose, then pump this simple sugar into our bloodstream. Some glucose is immediately used to power our cells, and some gets stored in our muscles or liver to be used later. Any remaining glucose is turned into fat and stockpiled in special fat storage cells.

How many calories do Canadians consume?

The average Canadian consumes about 2,780 calories per day. That's about 400 calories more than what the average person consumed in 1991.

Health experts point to this steady increase of daily calorie consumption as one of the reasons so many Canadians are fighting with their weight. According to Statistics Canada, nearly one-quarter of adult Canadians are obese and an additional 35% are overweight. In total, that's 14.1 million Canadians.

How do calories influence healthy weight?

We all know that consuming more calories than our bodies can burn each day will likely lead to weight gain. And, conversely, that consuming fewer calories will lead to weight loss.

It's a simple equation—in theory. In real life, maintaining a healthy weight—and especially losing weight—can be quite complicated. That's why hundreds of researchers around the world are investigating the finer points of the formula. But the general rule of thumb is this: If you want to lose a pound a week—the amount health experts suggest is a healthy rate—you need to subtract 500 calories a day from your diet. The calories can be cut by either eating less or exercising more or a combination of the two.

How many calories does my body need for a healthy weight?

Your age, size, muscle mass and activity level all determine how many calories you need each day to maintain a healthy weight.

According to Canada's Food Guide, the average man, depending on his age and activity level, needs between 2,500 and 3,000 calories a day, while the average woman needs between 1,500 and 2,300 calories a day.

MEGAN'S TIP: It's been years since I worried about losing weight. For the most part, I'm happy with my current size. (If you don't know me, I am not, have never been and will never be a size 2. Or 4, or 6 . . .) Rather, my main concern these days is to avoid *gaining* weight—because putting on additional pounds will put me at greater risk for disease. Two long-term Harvard studies have shown middle-aged men and women who gained between 11 and 22 pounds after age 20 were up to three times as likely to develop heart disease, high blood pressure and type 2 diabetes as those who gained 5 pounds or less. Thwarting those diseases is my main incentive for keeping close to my college weight.

It all adds up

It's the little things that can help a lot when it comes to maintaining a healthy weight. Consuming an extra 100 calories a day can add up to about 10 pounds of weight gain in one year. It's a rather frightening thought. But you can use this fact to your favour. There are many ways to shave off 100 calories each day. Skipping the butter on your morning toast will get you about halfway there (1 tablespoon of butter is 100 calories). Ditching your can-a-day pop habit will cut out 150 calories each day for a weekly savings of 1,000 calories.

Take a good look at your snacks as well. Many Canadians get more of their calories from snacks than from breakfast. That's not a good thing if we are swapping oatmeal for oatmeal cookies.

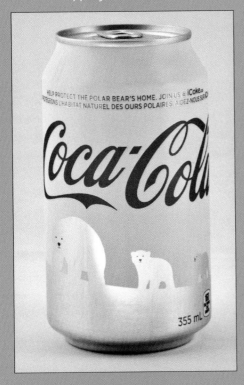

While we all like snacks—the average Canadian gets 23% of his or her daily calories from tidbits between meals—those who live on the east coast are the biggest snackers in the country. Atlantic Canadians get 26% of their calories from snacks. Quebec residents appear to have stronger willpower: snacks account for just 20% of their calories.

What does 100 calories look like?

It can be hard to picture the calories in our food, especially when stomachs are at their hungriest. To help, here is what 100 calories' worth of some of our favourite foods looks like.

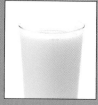

200 mL orange juice

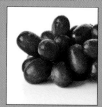

30 seedless grapes

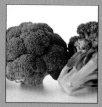

2 stalks of broccoli

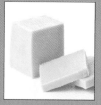

25 grams cheddar cheese

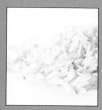

Scant 1/2 cup cooked rice

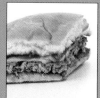

1/3 of a McDonald's cheeseburger

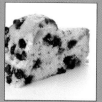

1/4 of a Tim Hortons chocolate-chip muffin

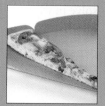

1/6 of a Pizza Pizza walk-in slice of Garden Veggie pizza

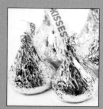

4 1/2 Hershey's Kisses

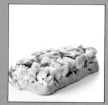

60% of a Nature Valley Sweet & Salty Granola Bar, peanut flavour

Why our bodies need fat

Why does my body need fat?

While we may resent the body fat that nestles around our hips and bellies, dietary fat is an important macronutrient for our bodies. Along with providing fuel to our cells, fat (and its sidekick, cholesterol) is a raw material for making cell membranes. Fat is also used in the coatings around nerve fibres and is a building block for some hormones. Without fat in our diets, our bodies would not be able to absorb important vitamins, such as vitamins A, E and D.

How does my body use fat?

Our bodies break down the fat we consume into smaller pieces of fat. To help them move through the bloodstream (just as oil doesn't dissolve in water, fat can't dissolve in blood), our bodies cover the broken-up bits of fat with protein. These particles come in different sizes and densities.

Triglycerides are the main way our bodies transport fat and are important for good health. But researchers have linked an excess of triglycerides circulating in the bloodstream to heart disease, stroke and diabetes. Making sure you don't consume more calories than your body requires will help lower your risk of developing unhealthy levels of triglycerides.

High-density lipoprotein, or HDL, is commonly called the "good" cholesterol because it hunts down the bad cholesterol in the bloodstream and takes it to the liver for disposal. This cholesterol cleaning service helps to prevent arteries from becoming clogged and is why having a high level of HDL is associated with good heart health.

Low-density lipoprotein, or LDL, is known as the "bad" cholesterol. Too much LDL in the blood can lead to the buildup of plaque on the inner walls of arteries. Plaque deposits become dangerous when a blood clot gets caught in the narrowed artery, causing heart attack or stroke. If you have high LDL cholesterol, lowering it is one of the best ways to reduce your risk of heart disease and stroke.

How much fat should I consume each day?

Health experts suggest that between 20 and 35% of our daily calories should come from fat. For women, this means 45 to 75 grams a day. For men, it's 60 to 105 grams.

While sticking to these recommended daily intakes is important, the quality—or type—of fat we consume is more important than quantity when it comes to health.

Unsaturated fats: The good

Unsaturated fats improve cholesterol levels in the blood and are an important part of your daily diet. There are two main types of unsaturated fats: monounsaturated and polyunsaturated. Both improve blood cholesterol levels by lowering the LDL, or bad cholesterol, in our bodies.

Monounsaturated fats are found in high concentrations in plant oils, such as canola, peanut and olive oils, and in most nuts and seeds. Avocados are also a good source of this kind of fat.

Polyunsaturated fats are found in high concentrations in sunflower, corn and flaxseed oils and in foods such as walnuts, soybeans, pine nuts and cold-water fish.

Saturated fats: The bad

Consuming saturated fats increases the LDL—the "bad" cholesterol—in your blood. Too bad, because saturated fats are found in many tasty foods, including meat and animal fat (hamburgers, chicken wings), full-fat dairy products (ice cream) and some vegetable oils, including palm and coconut oil.

A good rule to follow is to choose unsaturated fats over saturated whenever possible.

Trans fats: The ugly

Trans fats are the villains of the food world. While small amounts are found in some animal-based foods, the majority of trans fats are of the man-made kind. These partially hydrogenated oils are the worst types of fats because they raise the bad cholesterol *and* lower the good cholesterol in the blood. They have no redeeming qualities—for health, that is.

Food manufacturers, on the other hand, have had a love affair with partially hydrogenated vegetable oils. Trans fats don't spoil as easily as other fats, they are easier to transport than liquid fats and they can be heated over and over again in a deep fryer.

Fried foods from fast-food outlets and prepackaged baked goods, including crackers, have traditionally been made with trans fats. In 2007, Canada asked the food industry to limit trans fats in its foods to less than 5% of the total fat content. But trans fats are still out there. It's up to you to check food labels and ask restaurants about the kinds of fats they use in the kitchen. If you see or hear the phrase "partially hydrogenated vegetable oil" or "partially hydrogenated shortening," steer clear. Most health experts say there is no safe amount of trans fats.

How much fat do Canadians consume?

Statistics Canada estimates about 25% of adult Canadians consume more fat than what experts recommend for good health. And the most recent Canadian Community Health Survey shows about 16% of the fat we consume comes from pizza, sandwiches, submarines, hamburgers and hot dogs. An additional 8% comes from sweet baked goods, such as cakes, cookies, muffins and doughnuts. That means at least one-quarter of the fat we consume is likely coming from unhealthy sources. Not good news for our arteries.

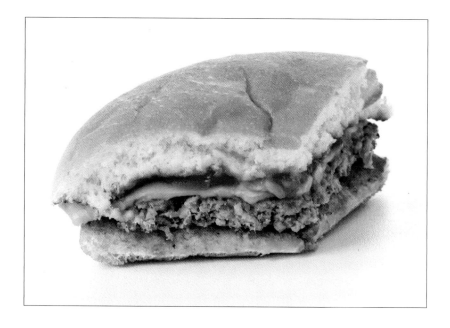

Essential eating

Essential fatty acids are called essential for a reason: the body needs them for critical functions, and it can't make them from scratch. Omega-3 fatty acids are an important type of essential fatty acid (omega-6s being the other kind). Omega-3s are polyunsaturated fats and true multi-taskers. Omega-3 fatty acids help to lower LDL—the "bad" cholesterol—in our blood and play a role in keeping our heart beating steadily. They are important for brain function and key to good growth and development. Some hormones couldn't be made without them. And the body also needs them to form cell membranes.

The easiest way to ensure you get enough omega-3 fatty acids in your diet is to eat two servings of fatty fish, such as salmon, herring or trout, each week. Next time you sit down to dinner at a restaurant, search the menu for a fish entree. Your heart and brain will thank you.

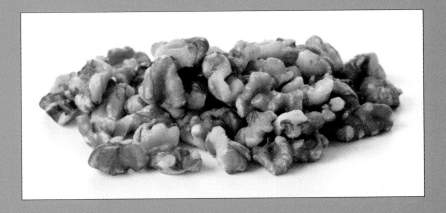

Why our bodies need sodium

What is sodium?

Sodium is an abundant metallic element found in the natural environment. You'll also find it listed in the periodic table. (If you paid attention during high school chemistry, you'll remember the symbol for sodium is Na. How often did that trip you up in quizzes?)

Some foods have a trace amount of naturally occurring sodium. An apple, for example, has 1 mg of sodium. But most of the sodium in our food has been added in the form of sodium chloride, more commonly known as table salt. Food manufacturers use salt to enhance the taste of their products, just as you sprinkle salt on your meal at home. They also rely on salt as a preservative and use it to influence the structure and texture of food.

Why does my body need sodium?

Sodium is essential for health. It helps transmit nerve impulses, it aids in muscle contraction and it's used, along with potassium, to maintain the right balance of fluids in our bodies. We need only a little sodium to perform these functions. When we consume too much it can be harmful to our health.

How much sodium do Canadians consume?

Each day, adult Canadians consume about 3,400 mg of sodium. That's much more than we need. The current consensus is that healthy adult Canadians need 1,500 mg of sodium a day. Adults over the age of 51 need 1,300 mg, while those over 71 need just 1,200 mg of sodium a day.

In our modern food environment, most of us easily surpass these recommended daily intakes. That's why Health Canada has also set an upper intake level of 2,300 mg of sodium a day. The best evidence shows this number is the highest average daily intake of sodium unlikely to cause health problems.

Why should I worry about consuming too much sodium?

When you have an excess amount of sodium in your body, it pulls water from cells into your bloodstream, thereby increasing blood pressure. Over time, an elevated blood pressure can cause health problems—a host of them.

High blood pressure is the major cause of cardiovascular disease, the number one cause of death in Canada, and a risk factor for stroke and kidney disease. Some research has also linked a diet high in sodium to osteoporosis, asthma and stomach cancer. According to the Heart and Stroke Foundation of Canada, reducing our daily sodium intake by 1,840 mg could save about 1 in 7 people dying from stroke and 1 in 11 people dying from coronary artery disease.

What can I do to cut back on sodium?

It would be nice if shelving the salt shaker were the only thing we needed to do to reduce our daily sodium intake. The problem is that about 77% of the sodium we consume each day comes from processed and prepackaged foods, and from the meals, snacks and beverages we consume outside our homes.

Just 11% of our sodium comes from the salt we use while cooking or from the small sprinkles we add to our meals, while 12% comes from the naturally occurring sodium found in foods. This means we need to carefully inspect food labels and scour nutrition facts provided by restaurants to ferret out which foods are high in sodium. We also need to limit the amount of processed foods we eat and choose more fresh foods to help cut sodium from our diets.

The bottom line is that it takes a lot of effort to consume a healthy amount of sodium—especially for those of us who frequently dine out.

MEGAN'S TIP: One simple way to cut salt when dining out is to order smaller portions or take half of your meal home. After spending hours poring over nutrition numbers, I've learned that one can easily consume twice the daily sodium limit in one meal out. Since I can't oversee the cook, I often take half my entree home to eat the following day for lunch. That way the saltiness is spread over two days. It's not a true sodium fix, but it does help.

THE SKINNY ON SALT: A thousand milligrams of sodium seems seriously salty. In fact, 1,200 mg is found in just 1/2 teaspoon of salt. Surprising, right? You can see how quickly sodium can add up.

Because it's hard to picture milligrams of sodium in your meals, I have translated the sodium content of featured foods into the equivalent number of dashes of salt from a traditional tabletop salt shaker. One dash of salt has about 40 mg of sodium.

Look for the salt shakes info in this book to quickly pinpoint a food's saltiness. Those with fewer than 10 salt shakes are considered low-sodium foods. And about 38 salt shakes is the amount of sodium your body needs in a day. I think you'll be surprised to see how much sodium is skulking in your favourite foods.

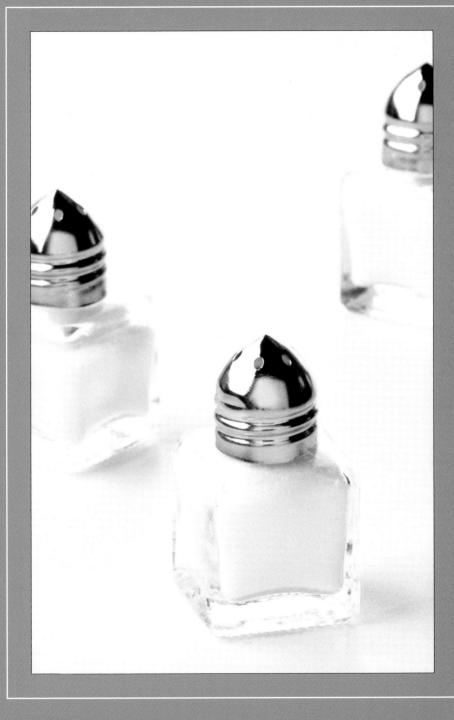

Why our bodies need carbohydrates

What are carbohydrates?

Carbohydrates are found in many foods and come in various forms. That oatmeal muffin you had for breakfast contains carbohydrates. So does the banana you had for a snack. Carbohydrates are also in your midday sandwich, in the pop you sipped while driving home from work and in the baked potato you ate alongside your steak at dinner.

The basic building block of every carbohydrate is a sugar molecule. How those molecules are put together determine the type of carbohydrate. The three main types—from a human nutrition standpoint—are sugars, starches and fibres.

Why does my body need carbohydrates?

Carbohydrates power every cell and system in the body. They are the body's main source of energy and are particularly important as fuel for the brain. Did you know it's the only organ in your body entirely dependent on carbohydrates for energy?

Carbohydrates (the apple kind, not the candy kind) also act as delivery vehicles, bringing essential vitamins and minerals and important phytonutrients into the body.

How does my body use carbohydrates?

The body turns most digestible carbohydrates into glucose, the sugar molecule used to power cells. Of the three main types of carbohydrates—sugars, starches and fibres—sugars are the easiest for the body to digest.

Many foods have added sugars. Others, such as fruits, have naturally occurring sugars—that's why they taste sweet. For the most part, the body quickly turns both kinds of sugars into glucose, which then flies through the bloodstream to power cells.

Starches, the kind of carbohydrate found in grains, potatoes, yams, corn and legumes, among other foods, also raise blood sugar levels. How quickly they are digested depends on the type of starch. Interestingly, a russet potato raises blood sugar levels quicker than a sweet potato.

The body has the hardest time digesting fibre. In fact, it can't. But fibre still has an important role to play in health.

How many carbohydrates should I consume each day?

On average, adult Canadians get about 50% of their daily calories from carbohydrates. That means most of us are doing pretty well: health experts suggest that 45 to 65% of our daily calories come from carbs. Depending on how many calories you consume, that works out to about 220 to 330 grams a day for men and 180 to 230 grams a day for women.

What kinds of carbohydrates are best to eat?

That straightforward question has a complicated answer. Books have been written on the subject, and dozens of researchers continue to parse out the finer details of which foods provide the best source of carbohydrates for human health. The current consensus (very briefly and very simply) is that harder-to-digest carbohydrates are a better choice than easily digestible carbs. A diet rich in easily digestible carbohydrates, such as those found in sweetened baked goods and breads and pastas made with refined flours, has been linked to an increased risk for obesity, heart disease and diabetes. Those found in fruits, vegetables and whole grains are considered to be "good" carbohydrates, so eating these types of foods is the best way to ensure you are looking after your health.

Most Canadians don't consume enough fruits and vegetables. Canada's Food Guide suggests women should aim for 7 to 8 servings and men 8 to 10 servings a day.

Not surprisingly, women do a better job than men of getting their daily dose of fruits and veggies. But don't go waving your salad fork in victory just yet, ladies. Recent surveys by Statistics Canada show that just 50% of women and 37% of men eat five or more servings a day

Why should I care about dietary fibre?

Unlike other forms of carbohydrates, fibre can't be broken down into sugar molecules by your body. But even though it passes through the body undigested, fibre does some important work as it travels the intestines.

Soluble fibre, which dissolves in water, is considered the heart-healthy kind because it scoops up fatty deposits as it moves through the intestines, taking them out of the body as waste. This helpful task lowers LDL cholesterol (the bad kind) and helps to regulate blood sugar levels. Oatmeal, nuts and seeds, beans and lentils and some fruits, including apples, strawberries and blueberries, are sources of soluble fibre.

Insoluble fibre, which does not dissolve in water, is considered the colon-friendly kind. It acts like a plow, pushing food through the intestinal tract, which promotes regularity and prevents constipation. Wheat bran, whole-grain breakfast cereals, whole-wheat bread, brown rice and some vegetables, including carrots, zucchini and tomatoes, are sources of insoluble fibre.

How much fibre should I consume each day?

Most Canadians eat only about half as much fibre as they need. Health experts recommend that women try to get 25 grams of fibre a day, while men should aim for about 38 grams.

To boost fibre intake, slowly add more fibre-rich foods to your diet. An easy way to start is to eat more fruits and vegetables. Raspberries, blackberries, corn and peas are very high in fibre, each with more than 4 grams per serving (one serving is a 1/2 cup). Including more whole grains, such as barley and bulgur, as well as beans and lentils in your meals is another simple way to get the benefits of fibre.

Why our bodies need protein

What is protein?

Proteins are made up of long chains of amino acids. Amazingly, there are at least 10,000 different proteins in the body. Each kind is composed of a unique sequence of amino acids.

Why does my body need protein?

Protein forms the major components of your organs, muscles, tendons and blood vessels, as well as of your skin and hair. Its most important job is to build, maintain and replace tissues in the body. But protein also has dozens of other critical functions. Some kinds help generate energy. Some make up the oxygen-carrying hemoglobin in the blood. Others are key players in the immune system.

To keep up with demand, your body has to constantly make new proteins from amino acids. Most amino acids can be produced in the body, but some are found only in protein-rich foods. This is why your body counts on a daily supply of dietary protein.

How much protein should I consume each day?

Health experts have determined that the average adult needs to consume 0.8 grams of protein for every kilogram of body weight. (Remember, 1 kilogram is equivalent to 2.2 pounds.) That means a person who weighs 150 pounds (68 kilograms) should eat about 55 grams of protein each day.

It's easy to use this simple formula to calculate your protein needs: multiply your weight in kilograms by 0.8. Or you can follow Health Canada guidelines, which recommend that women get 46 grams and men get 56 grams of protein each day.

There's really no need for worry here. Almost every one of us gets enough protein from our normal daily diet.

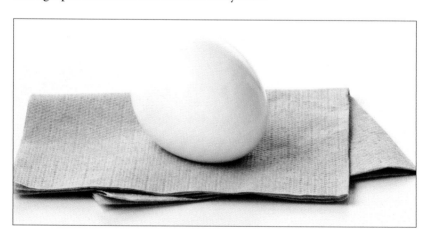

What are the best sources of protein for optimum health?

Although researchers have figured out the minimum amount of protein we need to keep our bodies running smoothly, they haven't yet determined how much—or what kind—of protein is best for our health. Until they have a definitive answer, a good general rule is to pay attention to what else comes packaged with your protein. For example, some high-protein foods—a tasty T-bone steak, say—are also high in saturated fat, while others—a broiled piece of salmon—deliver a dose of heart-healthy omega-3 fatty acids.

You can't go wrong if your protein choices are lean, well-trimmed cuts of meat, skinless poultry and fish that have been baked, broiled or grilled (dunking strips of chicken breast in a deep fryer negates their leanness). Vegetable sources of protein, such as beans, tofu, nuts and nut butters, are good choices, too.

Is all dietary protein created equal?

No, there are two kinds of dietary protein: complete and incomplete.

Complete protein contains all the amino acids your body needs to build new proteins. Meat, poultry, eggs, fish and dairy products tend to be good sources of complete protein.

Incomplete protein, most often found in plant-based sources, lacks some of the essential amino acids, those amino acids your body cannot produce from scratch. Vegetarians—well, all of us, really—need to eat a variety of foods every day to ensure that our bodies get the right amount and assortment of amino acids.

It's all about the plate

The easy way to eat well

While knowing some nutrition facts is undoubtedly helpful, many of us are looking for ways to simplify our busy lives. Health organizations have figured this out and have come up with a simple method to help people eat well. It requires just one tool, a plate. The idea is to fill one-quarter of your plate with protein, one-quarter with grains and the remainder with fruits and vegetables, the more colourful and varied, the better. Nutrition experts say that if you follow this method, you will end up ahead in the health department.

Now, some caveats: This method works as long as your plate isn't a size appropriate for giants. And it can be hard to follow at restaurants and drive-thrus because the portions served there are so large. It also takes some imagination with a sandwich or stir-fry or any other meal whose contents are piled together instead of spread out over the plate. The next few pages provide some ideas to help you get started.

What a good breakfast looks like at home

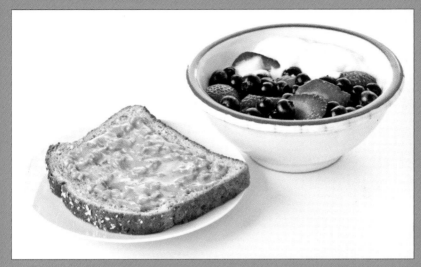

A slice of whole-grain bread, toasted, spread with 1 tablespoon of natural peanut butter. Enjoy with 1 cup of low-fat plain yogurt sprinkled with 1 cup of sliced strawberries and 1/2 a cup of blueberries.

What it looks like at Starbucks

Half of a toasted whole-grain bagel with peanut butter, a fruit cup and tall non-fat latte.

What it looks like at Tim Hortons

Homestyle Oatmeal with mixed berries and a small carton of low-fat milk. A piece of fruit and a handful of nuts from home will round out the meal.

What a good lunch looks like at home

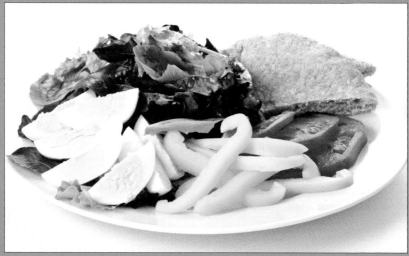

A salad made with 3 cups of mixed greens, topped with chopped tomato and sliced bell pepper and tossed with 2 tablespoons of light balsamic dressing. Round out the salad with half of a whole-wheat pita and two hard-boiled eggs.

What it looks like at the grocery store

Personal-sized grab-and-go salad with a light dressing (use no more than half a package) and two hard-boiled eggs with a small whole-grain roll from the bakery. A small carton of chocolate milk can be your treat.

What it looks like at McDonald's

A small green salad with light dressing (again, don't use more than half a package) and a Grilled Chicken Snack Wrap (get it without the creamy sauce to save calories). The Fruit 'n Yogurt Parfait can be your dessert.

What a good dinner looks like at home

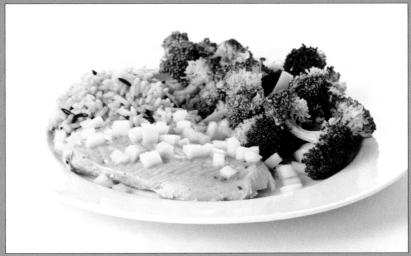

A piece of baked salmon (about the size of your palm) topped with a 1/4 cup of chopped mango and accompanied by a portion of brown rice pilaf (about the size of your fist) and roughly 1 1/2 cups of steamed vegetables (broccoli is my favourite).

What it looks like at Swiss Chalet

A Quarter Chicken Dinner with white meat, multigrain roll and side garden salad with dressing on the side. Use just a drizzle.

What it looks like at East Side Mario's

Spaghettini Bolognese from the Everyday Values menu (consider taking half or one-third of the entree home for lunch the next day) with a side of roasted vegetables.

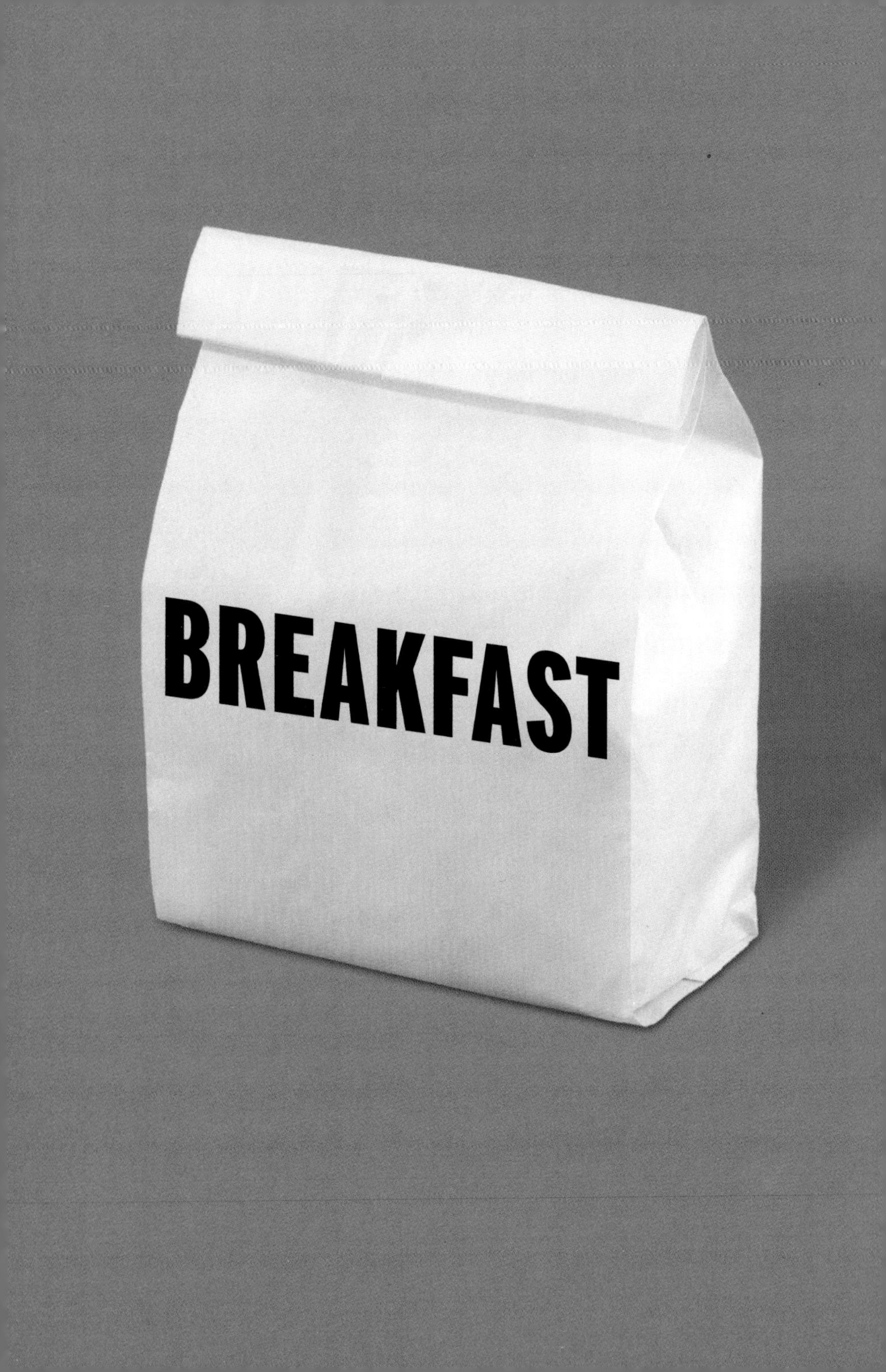
BREAKFAST

The age-old nutrition adage is spot-on: breakfast *is* the most important meal of the day. A good breakfast starts your metabolism off on the right track. My farmer ancestors knew this and began each morning with a plateful of eggs and meat, homemade bread with fruit preserve, potatoes, beans, pancakes with syrup and maybe even a piece of pie to fill in any remaining spaces in their stuffed-to-the-gills stomachs. All to fuel them through seven hours of back-breaking manual labour.

These days, most of us push paper, not plows. But we still need a breakfast that will sustain us through the morning. Just not a farmhouse feast.

What to look for in a breakfast

Most modern-day breakfasts are packed with sugar and highly refined carbohydrates. Sweetened cereals, cake-like muffins, fluffy bagels—all of these popular choices are quick-hit foods. They taste good and give you a spurt of energy but burn out before you get much benefit.

It's important to start the day with a breakfast that won't disappear from your belly before you pull into the office. A nourishing morning meal will reduce mid-morning cravings, boost energy levels and increase concentration. And it will make it more likely you'll eat a sensible lunch.

Look for a breakfast that has

Good-quality protein. This will help keep hunger at bay all morning. It could be a small handful of chopped nuts on your cereal. A tablespoon of natural nut butter on your whole-grain toast. A hard-boiled egg. Or a bowl of yogurt.

Whole grains. These slow-burning carbs won't send you on the sugar rush and crash delivered by foods made with refined carbohydrates. When choosing cereal or bread, look for brands whose first ingredient is a whole grain.

Along with smoothing out hunger peaks, adding whole grains to your morning meal will help reduce the risk of heart attack. As well, whole grains are packed with vitamins, heart-healthy phytonutrients and fibre that aids with digestion.

Whole fruit instead of juice. An orange has half the calories of orange juice, and it offers much more fibre for roughly the same amount of vitamin C. Keep a bowl of fruit near the door so you can grab a piece when you leave in the morning. Fresh fruit almost never appears in takeout breakfast meals.

Limit breakfast foods that have

Processed meats. Research has linked processed meats such as sausage, bacon and ham to an increased risk of diabetes and cancer, particularly colorectal cancer. The Canadian Cancer Society suggests saving processed meats for special occasions.

Lots of sugar. Sweetened cereals, breakfast pastries, doughnuts, most muffins and even white bread are foods that quickly enter the bloodstream, which leaves you feeling hungry within just a few hours of eating.

Humongous portions. You don't want to use up all of your daily allotment of calories before lunch.

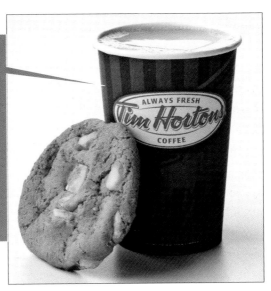

A double-double can be trouble-trouble. A medium Tim's coffee with two creams and two sugars has 230 calories and 12 grams of fat. It's like drinking a white-chocolate macadamia-nut cookie.

You can save 100 calories and 10 grams of fat by just switching to a double-double with milk.

McDonald's Egg McMuffin

The Egg McMuffin is the original fast-food breakfast. Before it was rolled out, in the mid-1970s, people had to sit down at a table to eat their bacon and eggs. McDonald's revolutionized breakfast by creating the first morning meal people could eat on the go. It was an instant hit, and the classic still satisfies thousands every morning.

With a sensible 290 calories and a sustaining dose of belly-filling protein, the Egg McMuffin remains one of the best breakfasts you can get at a drive-thru window.

Calories: 290
Fat: 12 grams
Carbohydrates: 29 grams
Protein: 16 grams
Sodium: 760 mg
Salt shakes: 19

DANGER ZONE: Resist the Sausage, Egg & Cheese McGriddles. The sweetened bread with sausage, egg and cheese has 550 calories, 30 grams of fat and 1,430 mg of sodium. You would do better downing a McDonald's cheeseburger and a small order of fries.

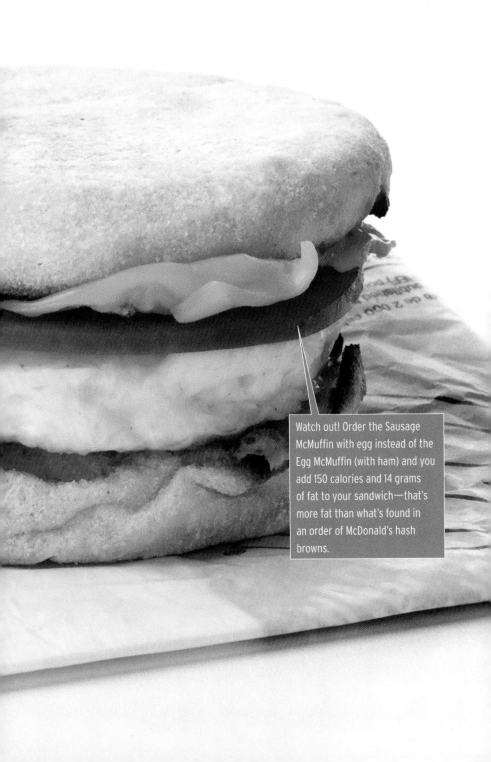

Watch out! Order the Sausage McMuffin with egg instead of the Egg McMuffin (with ham) and you add 150 calories and 14 grams of fat to your sandwich—that's more fat than what's found in an order of McDonald's hash browns.

Tim Hortons Homestyle Biscuit with sausage, egg and cheese

This palm-sized meal has the highest fat content of any Timmies breakfast sandwich. Unless you want to be eating greens the rest of the day, consider skipping the sandwich made with sausage. It contains about half of your day's worth of fat.

Calories: 530
Fat: 34 grams
Carbohydrates: 36 grams
Protein: 19 grams
Sodium: 1,010 mg
Salt shakes: 25

SMART SWAP: The best bet? Order the Egg White Omelette Breakfast Sandwich with ham, cheese and a whole-grain English muffin. You'll get the warm gooey goodness of a breakfast sandwich for only 240 calories, 7 grams of fat and 830 mg of sodium. Plus you'll get two additional grams of fibre.

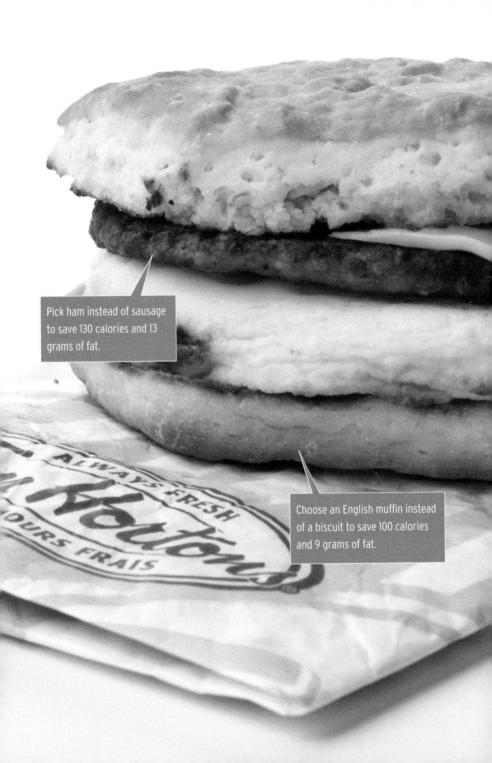

Fries for breakfast?

Using the term "hash browns" helps to hide the fact that this popular breakfast side is nothing more than deep-fried potato. Sure they're yummy, but do you really need to eat fried, salted spuds before your neurons are fully functioning? If you skip the hash browns at your next fast-food breakfast, you will have at least an extra 100 calories in your daily calorie budget.

McDonald's hash browns

An order of McDonald's hash browns weighs 16 grams less than a small order of fries. But this small potato patty has about the same amount of fat *and* 190 mg more sodium.

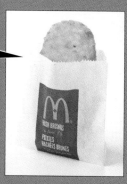

Calories: 160

Fat: 10 grams

Carbohydrates: 16 grams

Protein: 1 gram

Sodium: 360 mg

Salt shakes: 9

Tim Hortons hash browns

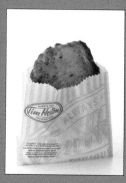

Calories: 100

Fat: 5 grams

Carbohydrates: 12 grams

Protein: 1 gram

Sodium: 210 mg

Salt shakes: 5

HOW MUCH FAT'S IN THAT?

Burger King hash browns look, smell and taste like french fries but they may be fattier than you think.

1 medium order of Burger King hash browns

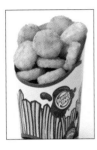

Calories: 450
Fat: 30 grams
Carbohydrates: 42 grams
Protein: 4 grams
Sodium: 660 mg
Salt shakes: 16 1/2

EQUALS

15 Honey Dip Timbits

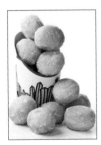

Calories: 900
Fat: 30 grams
Carbohydrates: 135 grams
Protein: 15 grams
Sodium: 750 mg
Salt shakes: 19

A medium order of BK hash browns has as much fat as 15 Honey Dip Timbits.

Cora 1990's Harvest

French toast made with cinnamon-raisin brioche and topped with three strips of bacon, an egg and "a mountain" of fresh fruit is one of Cora's most popular dishes. Its heft is impressive. It's sort of like getting a whole breakfast buffet on a plate.

On the plus side, this meal has about three servings of fresh fruit, something Canadians don't get enough of every day. Unfortunately, the mound of fruit doesn't make up for the mound of calories on the other side of the plate.

Its 1,320 calories is about half of what the average man needs in a day, which makes this one-plate meal more like a breakfast, a morning snack and lunch combined.

Calories: 1,320
Fat: 46 grams
Carbohydrates: 195 grams
Protein: 31 grams
Sodium: 880 mg
Salt shakes: 22

MEGAN'S TIP: This is one of those meals that I split in two. Divvying it up—either with my dining companion or in a takeout container—means I get a generous piece of French toast, a bite or two of scrambled egg and a salty slice of bacon (eating just one piece, instead of three, saves about 6 grams of fat and almost 400 mg of sodium). With all the fresh fruit, I know I won't go hungry. Since the brioche is so sweet, and chopped fruit is the ideal topping on French toast, I also skip the butter and pancake syrup, to save about 200 calories and 11 grams of fat.

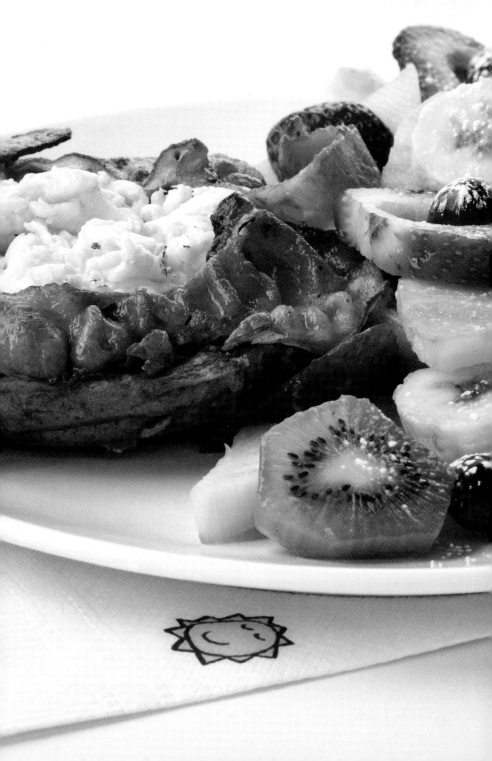

Tim Hortons bagel with cream cheese

During the low-fat dieting craze of the 1990s, the humble bagel burst onto the dining scene as the go-to guiltless meal. While the bagel may be low in fat, it can contain a surprising number of calories and, depending on its size, be the equivalent of five slices of bread. The Timmies sesame seed bagel with plain cream cheese runs to a substantial 414 calories.

Calories: 414
Fat: 16.5 grams
Carbohydrates: 55 grams
Protein: 12 grams
Sodium: 609 mg
Salt shakes: 15

SMART SWAP: Consider switching out the sesame seed bagel for the wheat 'n honey. It won't cut calories, but it will add a gram of fibre—something most Canadians don't get enough of every day.

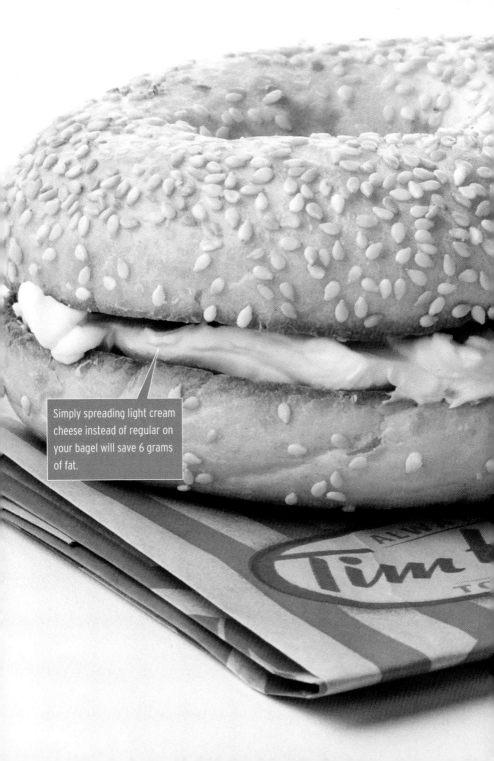

Simply spreading light cream cheese instead of regular on your bagel will save 6 grams of fat.

Tim Hortons Homestyle Oatmeal with mixed berries

The next time you pull into Tim Hortons for your morning meal, think about swapping out that muffin or sausage sandwich for a cup of takeout oatmeal. This humble breakfast, which Timmies slow cooks and makes with a few simple ingredients, has all the right components for a healthy start to the day. It is low in calories and fat, and the oatmeal provides 5 grams of fibre, about one-fifth of the average woman's daily needs.

Serving size: small

Calories: 210

Fat: 2.5 grams

Carbohydrates: 44 grams (including 14 grams sugars; 5 grams fibre)

Protein: 6 grams

Sodium: 220 mg

Salt shakes: 5 1/2

BREAKFAST BOOSTER: Drink a small carton of skim milk with your oatmeal to add 88 calories and 9 more grams of hunger-busting protein.

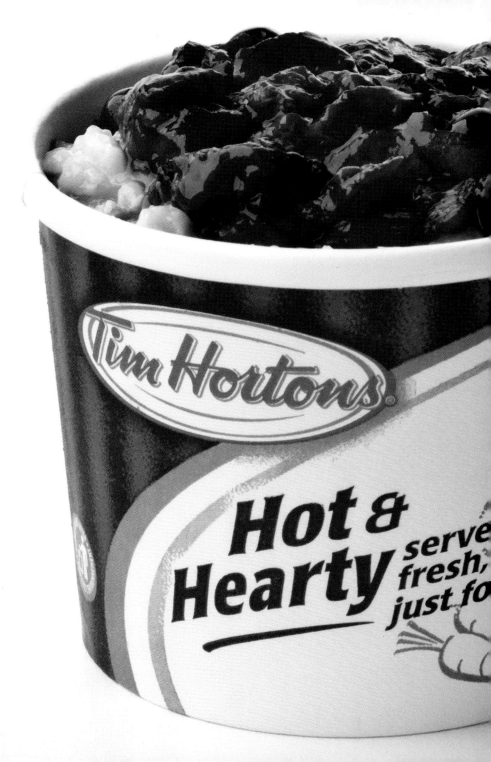

Tim Hortons blueberry muffin

This muffin has more sugar—the equivalent of 6 teaspoons—than almost any doughnut at Timmies. If you must have a blueberry muffin, choose the whole-grain version. Although it has 380 calories and 15 grams of fat, you get some nutritional benefit from the whole grains and its additional 3 grams of fibre.

Serving size: 115 grams

Calories: 340

Fat: 11 grams

Carbohydrates: 53 grams (including 25 grams sugars; 2 grams fibre)

Protein: 5 grams

Sodium: 570 mg

Salt shakes: 14

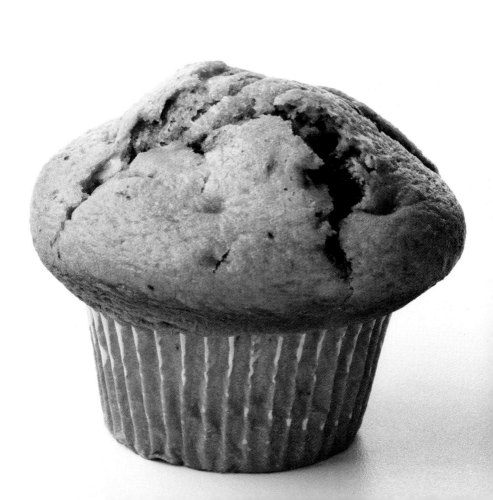

McDonald's blueberry muffin

A blueberry muffin sounds like a much healthier choice than a muffin made with chocolate and bits of cookie. But at McDonald's, the double chocolate muffin with Oreo crumble (which is more cupcake than muffin) has just 40 more calories than the blueberry version and the same amount of fat—a surprising fact that highlights the cupcakey-ness of the blueberry muffin.

Serving size: 121 grams

Calories: 410

Fat: 15 grams

Carbohydrates: 63 grams (including 33 grams sugars; 2 grams fibre)

Protein: 6 grams

Sodium: 320 mg

Salt shakes: 8

SMART SWAP: Love McDonald's muffins? Choose the golden bran and raisin version or the Fruit 'n Fibre for their whole grains and the added 4 to 6 grams of fibre. Might as well get some nutritional benefit for all those calories.

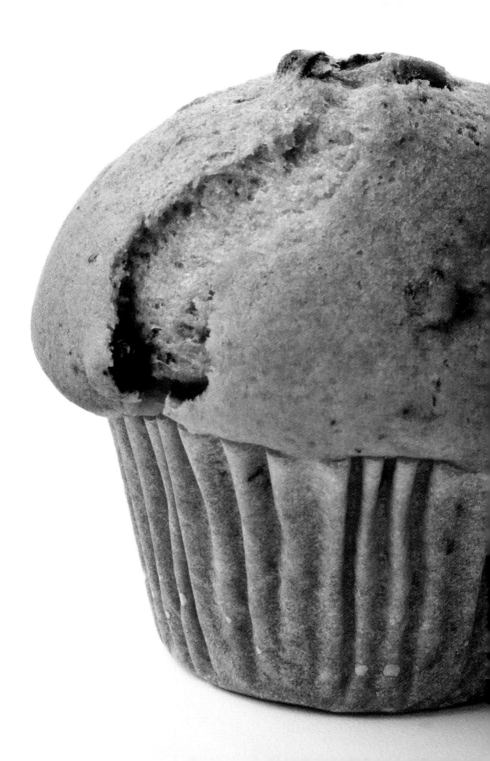

Costco blueberry muffin

This oversize muffin has roughly one-third of your day's worth of calories, half your daily fat allotment and more than half of the sodium your body needs in a day.

You can't buy just one muffin at Costco. You have to buy two packs of six. That's 7,644 calories in muffins. The best bet here is to split each muffin into halves (preferably into thirds) to rectify the warehouse-sized portion.

Serving size: 176 grams
Calories: 637
Fat: 34 grams
Carbohydrates: 73 grams
Protein: 10 grams
Sodium: 862 mg
Salt shakes: 21 1/2

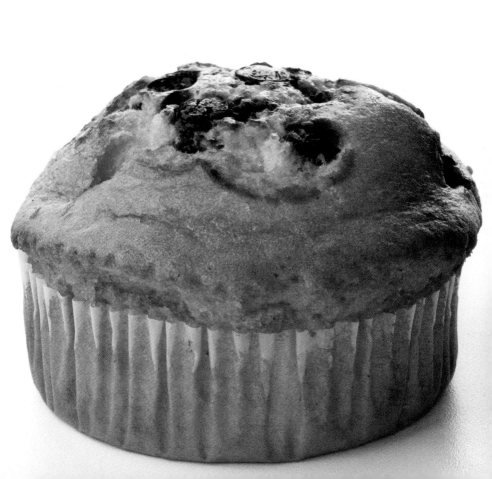

Sobeys blueberry muffin

One of the smaller muffins you'll find outside your home. This is a good thing. (A handy tip for spotting properly proportioned muffins: Look for ones about the size of a lemon.)

Instead of this six-pack of muffins, consider buying a half-dozen small whole-grain buns for the week. Eat them each morning with a smear of natural peanut butter and some sliced bananas.

Serving size: 105 grams
Calories: 310
Fat: 11 grams
Carbohydrates: 48 grams (including 23 grams sugars; 1 gram fibre)
Protein: 5 grams
Sodium: 290 mg
Salt shakes: 7

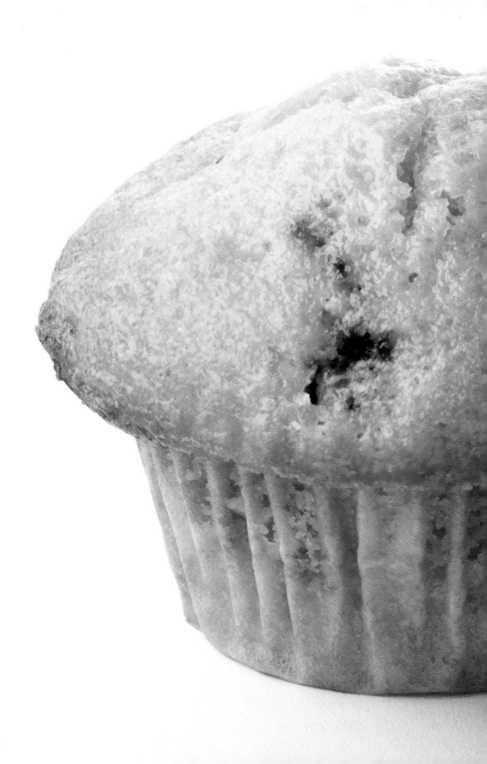

Apple banana berry muffins

Usually, I satisfy a muffin craving by baking a batch of fruit-filled whole-grain muffins at home. In just 45 minutes —that's 15 minutes of tinkering in the kitchen and 30 minutes of oven time—I have 12 high-fibre, low-fat, nutrient-rich muffins that can be popped into the freezer to eat for breakfast or as a hearty snack throughout the week. And yes, they taste good!

Here is a low-fat muffin recipe that I make over and over. The muffins taste great with a dollop of honey or jam. Feel free to sprinkle them with raw sugar instead of sliced almonds, and to use raspberries, chopped strawberries or blueberries.

1/2 cup plain non-fat yogurt
1/4 cup quick-cooking rolled oats
  (not instant)
1 cup fresh or frozen berries of
  your choice
1 1/4 cups plus 2 teaspoons
  whole-wheat flour
1 1/2 teaspoons baking powder
1 teaspoon baking soda

1/2 teaspoon salt
3/4 cup mashed ripe bananas
  (about 2)
3/4 cup unsweetened applesauce
2 large eggs, lightly beaten
2 tablespoons honey
1 teaspoon almond extract
1/4 cup sliced almonds

Preheat the oven to 375°F. Spray a 12-cup muffin tin with non-stick spray.

In a small bowl, mix the yogurt with the oats and set aside for about 5 minutes, or until oats are slightly softened.

In a small bowl, toss blueberries with 2 teaspoons of whole-wheat flour to coat.

In a medium-sized bowl, mix the remaining whole-wheat flour with the baking powder, baking soda and salt.

In a large bowl, combine bananas, applesauce, eggs, honey and almond extract. Add in the yogurt-oat mixture, stirring to combine.

Fold dry ingredients into the wet mixture and stir just until combined. Gently fold in the berries. Spoon batter into prepared muffin tin and sprinkle with the sliced almonds. Bake for 25 to 30 minutes. Cool on a wire rack. Makes 12.

Per muffin
Calories: 115
Fat: 2 grams
Carbohydrates: 21 grams (including 3 grams fibre)
Protein: 4 grams
Sodium: 220 mg
Salt shakes: 5 1/2

Recipe adapted with permission from *Moosewood Restaurant Cooking for Health*, by the Moosewood Collective.

Breakfast at the diner

The classic Canadian breakfast is a staple of diners, brunch bars and greasy spoons across the country. It's one of those weekend comforts we all love. Maybe it's the luxury of having someone else cook. No matter whether this favourite breakfast is the centre point of a family celebration or a cozy tête-à-tête the morning after spending a night with a new squeeze, revealing the nutrition numbers won't steer people away. But it is good to know what you are digging into so early in the day.

At Wimpy's Diner

The dish: Peameal bacon and eggs
What you get: Four pieces of peameal-style bacon with three eggs over easy, two pieces of toasted and buttered rye and a pile of home fries.
The verdict: This big breakfast clocks in with 969 calories, 50 grams of fat and 2,223 mg of sodium. That's about half your daily calories and more than half your daily fat. The salt-laden meal also brings you just shy of the maximum recommended daily sodium allowance.

Calories: 969
Fat: 50 grams
Carbohydrates: 79 grams
Protein: 51 grams
Sodium: 2,223 mg
Salt shakes: 55 1/2

Megan's Tip: I have to be awfully hungry to take on a big diner breakfast. When I do, I ask for the toast to come unbuttered and replace the hash browns (well, maybe just half) with fruit or tomato slices. These two tiny requests can save up to 10 grams of fat.

At Denny's

The dish: The Grand Slam

What you get: Hungry diners get to pick four items from a long list of breakfast favourites. A Grand Slam made with two scrambled eggs, two pieces of bacon, two slices of toast and a mound of hash browns is likely to be one of the more popular combinations.

The verdict: With its 810 calories, 54 grams of fat and 1,490 mg of sodium, Denny's classic breakfast combo brings a lot to the table—and all before lunch.

For a large man, the meal has a third of his daily calories, half his fat and almost all the sodium his body needs in a day.

Calories: 810

Fat: 54 grams

Carbohydrates: 60 grams

Protein: 28 grams

Sodium: 1,490 mg

Salt shakes: 37

Danger Zone: The Meat Lover's Scramble at Denny's has 1,130 calories, 66 grams of fat and an astonishing 3,180 mg of sodium. That's two eggs scrambled with bacon, diced ham and crumbled sausage, topped with cheddar cheese, and served with two strips of bacon, two sausage links and two buttermilk pancakes.

For men, this monstrous meal has half their daily calories, more than two-thirds of their fat and 38% more sodium than the maximum recommended daily amount.

Homemade diner breakfast

Don't get discouraged about diner breakfasts. All you need to do is by-pass the actual diner and cook up a plate of eggs and toast at home.

A homemade breakfast with 2 poached eggs, 2 strips of reduced-sodium bacon, 2 pieces of whole-wheat toast, 1/2 a tablespoon of marga-rine and 1 tablespoon of jam will have half the calories, half the fat and half the sodium of just about anything you'll find in a greasy spoon.

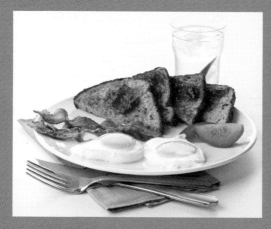

Calories: 537
Fat: 25 grams
Carbohydrates: 47 grams
Protein: 29 grams
Sodium: 900 mg
Salt shakes: 22 1/2

Megan's Tip: Many of us don't think of breakfast as a time to eat our veggies. But if you have time to whip up a plate of eggs at home, consider adding some seasonal vegetables to the meal. Maybe some steamed asparagus with a squeeze of lemon or pan-fried mushrooms or cherry tomatoes.

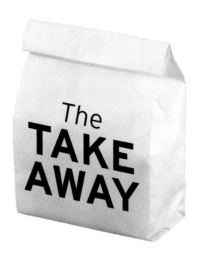

The
**TAKE
AWAY**

Build a breakfast that will power you through the morning.

Include good-quality protein such as a small handful of nuts, a poached egg or a cup of low-fat yogurt. You'll also need the high-quality carbohydrates found in whole grains.

Watch out for processed meats. A slice of ham, a strip of bacon or a sausage patty will add considerable calories, fat and sodium to your meal. Cancer experts recommend limiting these meats.

Beware the hash browns. Do you need to eat french fries for breakfast?

Don't have dessert for breakfast. Cake-like muffins and icing-covered pastries will leave you feeling hungry soon after eating.

Split the big sit-down breakfast. Eating half your day's calories before mid-morning will only slow you down.

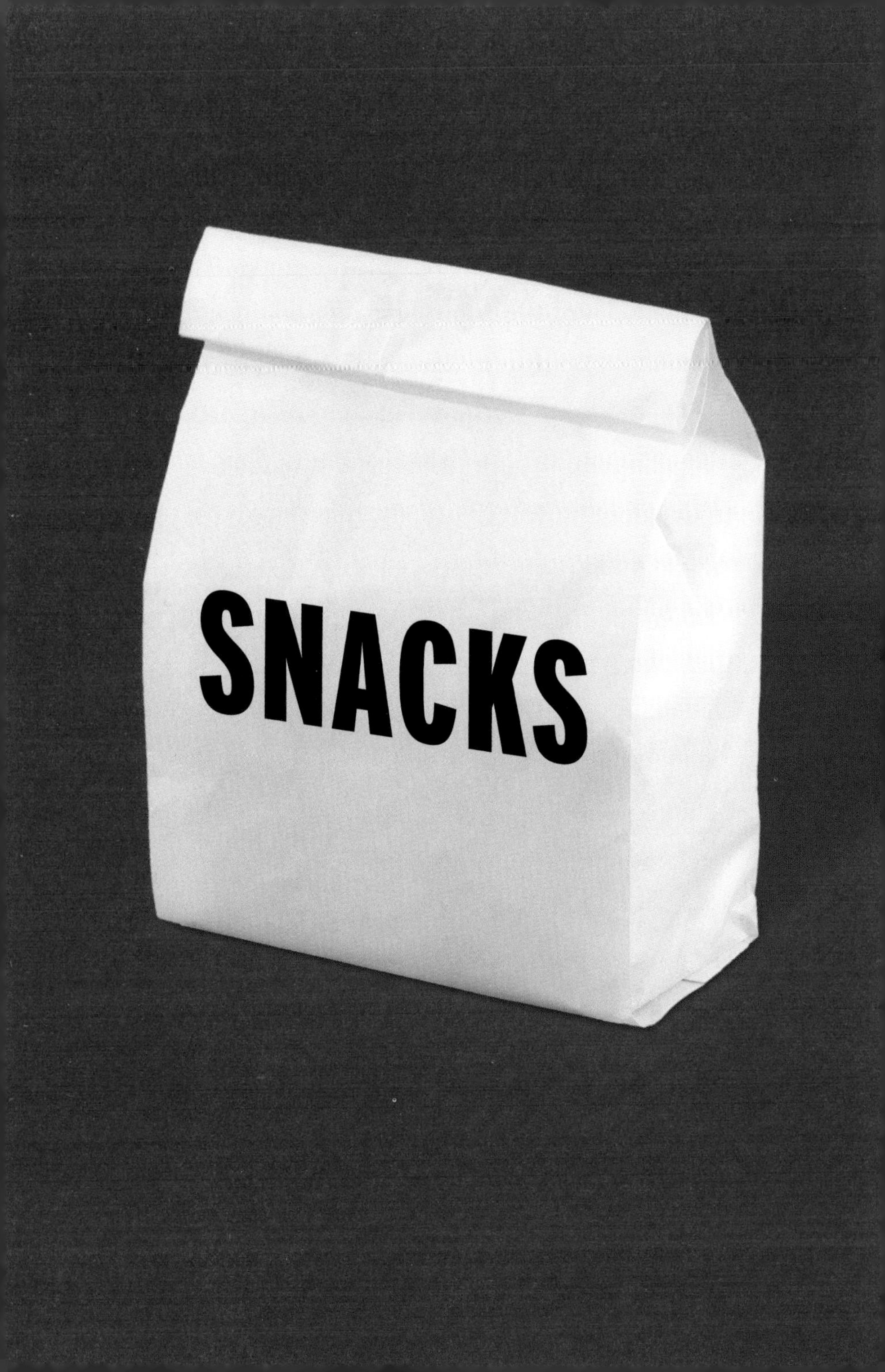
SNACKS

If you're driving down the highway rather than sitting at the dinner table, it's a whole lot easier to convince yourself that the calories you consume don't count—that the carton of chocolate milk or bag of chips aren't really part of your day.

In fact, when snacking away from home, it's easy to consume more calories than are in a meal. We tend to grab whatever is available when hunger hits, letting stomach grumbles dictate our food choices. It doesn't help that snacks are typically the size of mini-meals. And usually, when we munch on snacks, we do so mindlessly. Recall the time you popped mouthful after mouthful of potato chips, then were surprised to find you'd finished the entire bag.

When it comes to snacking, none of these things bode well for waistlines. The solution is to become a strategic snacker.

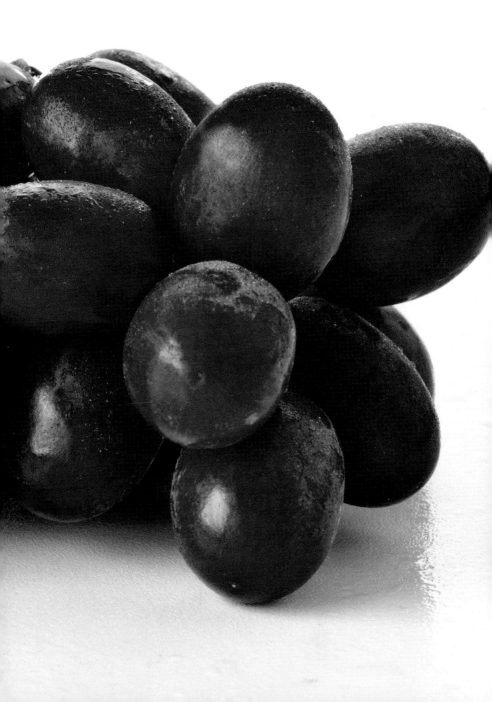

Why are you snacking?

Before you reach for a snack, ask yourself a few simple questions.

Am I thirsty?

Mild dehydration can feel like hunger pangs. So drink a glass of water (not pop!) and see if that helps to quiet your stomach.

Am I really hungry or am I just bored?

The workday blues can prompt some mindless snacking. If you want a mini-break from the keyboard, look for a low-calorie snack that takes a lot of chewing—maybe baby carrots with a fat-free dip or a couple of cups of air-popped popcorn and 10 almonds or a small handful of pretzel sticks. A brisk walk around the office may also lift the doldrums.

Am I hungry or am I simply tired?

If you think a snack will give you a much-needed boost of energy, opt for one packed with protein, not sugar. A hard-boiled egg, a palmful of nuts or a small glass of low-fat chocolate milk will do the trick.

Is this a snack or a mini-meal?

As workdays get longer and evening chores crowd the dinner hour, it's easy to get caught before supper needing a snack. You need something to quell those hunger pangs. But it can be hard to find a sensible snack under 500 calories, especially if it includes a sugary drink. Choose wisely—or split your snack—aiming for somewhere between 100 and 200 calories.

Petro-Canada: Rockstar energy drink and Twix cookie bar

Hungry and tired, with a long stretch of highway still ahead, you pull into a gas station to get an energy drink and something sweet at the convenience store. The can and candy bar look fairly inoffensive, but before you get far down the highway, you will have consumed 530 calories—about a quarter of what the average person needs in a day. And the 86 grams of sugar contained in this dual snack is like eating 20 teaspoons of sugar. Sure, you will be buzzing, but a sugar crash won't be far behind.

ROCKSTAR ENERGY DRINK

Serving size: 473 mL can

Calories: 280

Carbohydrates: 62 grams
   (all sugars)

Sodium: 80 mg

Salt shakes: 2

TWIX COOKIE BAR

Serving size: 2 cookie bars

Calories: 250

Fat: 12 grams

Carbohydrates: 33 grams
   (including 24 grams sugars;
   1 gram fibre)

Protein: 2 grams

Sodium: 100 mg

Salt shakes: 2 1/2

SMART SWAP: Instead of downing an energy drink, sip on coffee with milk. A small coffee contains about 179 mg of caffeine, while the typical energy drink has between 70 and 160 mg of caffeine. This simple switch will ensure you still get that caffeine kick-start. But you'll do it without the 15 teaspoons of sugar swimming in the energy drink.

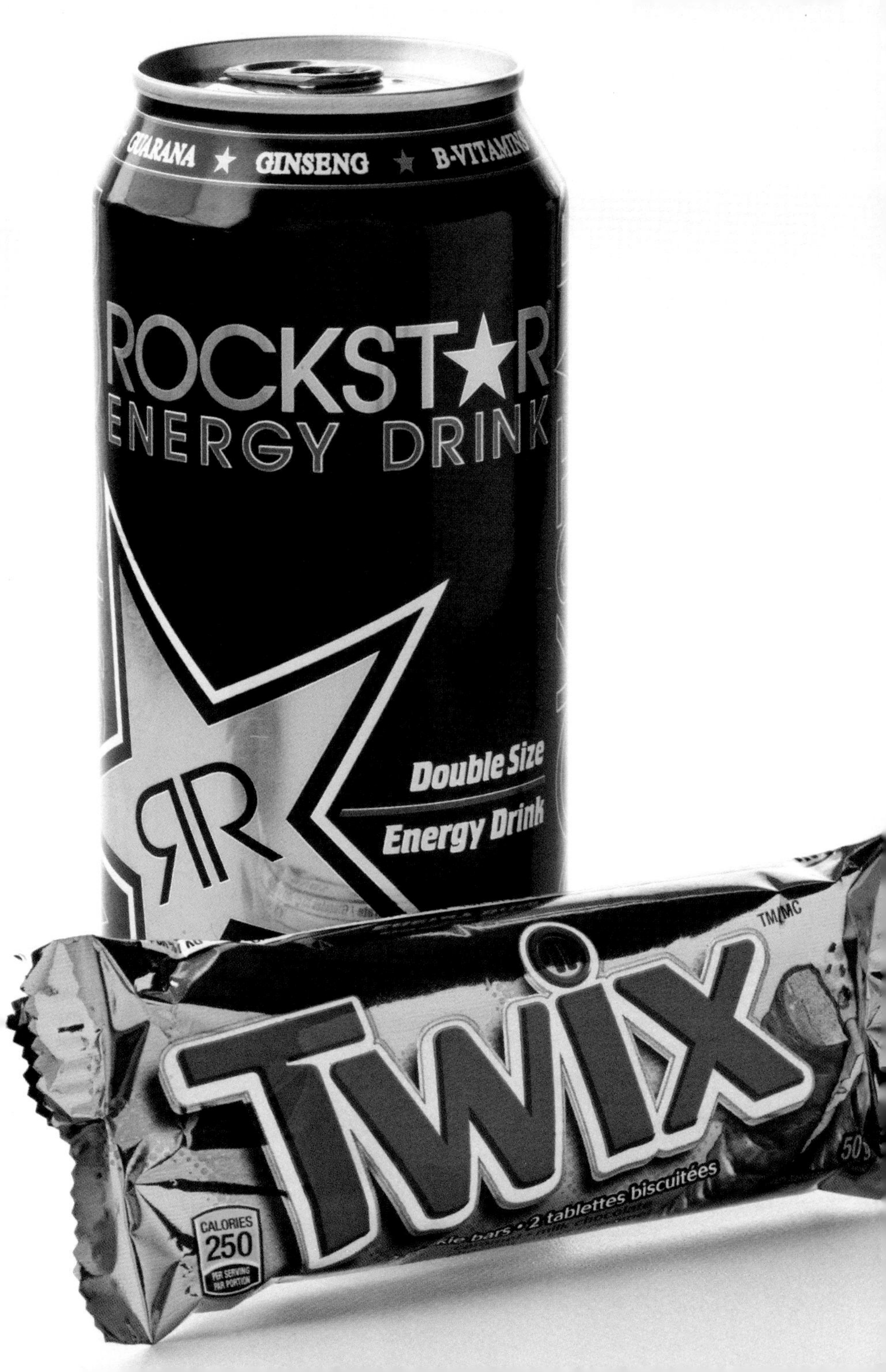
GUARANA ★ GINSENG ★ B-VITAMINS
ROCKSTAR
ENERGY DRINK
Double Size
Energy Drink
TM/MC
Twix
50g
2 tablettes biscuitées
CALORIES
250
PER SERVING
PAR PORTION

ESSO: PEP 'N CHED AND LAY'S CHIPS

Gas stations provide only three choices of fuel for your car. But the teeming snack aisles inside their convenience stores offer a boundless array of chips, cookies, crackers and candy. It can be tricky to find something that will settle your craving and be good for your waistline.

Grabbing a Pep 'n Ched and a bag of Lay's salt and vinegar chips at an Esso On the Run is hazardous. Together, the two items have more sodium than your body needs in a day. If that doesn't get you, consider that the combined 53 grams of fat is like consuming a dozen classic chicken wings from Pizza Pizza.

You—well, your body, at least—will notice the calories, fat and sodium skulking in these snacks.

PEP 'N CHED

Calories: 320

Fat: 27 grams

Carbohydrates: 1 gram

Protein: 18 grams

Sodium: 920 mg

Salt shakes: 23

LAY'S SALT AND VINEGAR CHIPS

Serving size: 75 grams

Calories: 400

Fat: 26 grams

Carbohydrates: 39 grams

Protein: 4 grams

Sodium: 670 mg

Salt shakes: 40

SORT OF SMART SWAPS: If you are craving something salty, just pick one—not two—of these snacks. And hunt for a smaller bag of chips or a shorter pepperoni stick (without the cheese). Even better, pick up a bag of sunflower seeds instead. The protein in the seeds will curb your hunger. And 1 cup of seeds has 315 calories—less than half that of the pepperoni and chips.

Pep 'n Ched and Lay's salt and vinegar chips

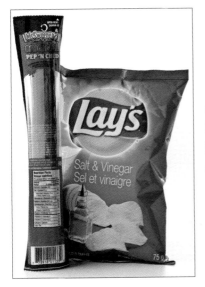

A Pep 'n Ched with a bag of Lay's salt and vinegar chips have as many calories as four grilled cheese sandwiches.

EQUALS

4 grilled cheese sandwiches

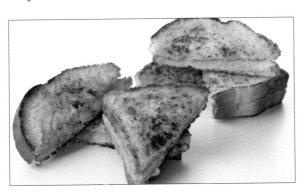

Mac's: Juici Jamaican-style spicy beef patty

This beef-filled patty may go down like a snack, but really, it's more like a mini-meal. It has about the same number of calories as Subway's 6-inch teriyaki chicken with sweet onion sub and three times more fat.

With 370 calories, it won't break the belly bank, but don't pull into a drive-thru an hour later for lunch.

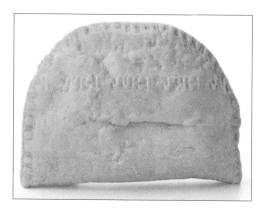

Calories: 370
Fat: 15 grams
Carbohydrates: 47 grams
Protein: 12 grams
Sodium: 620 mg
Salt shakes: 15 1/2

SMART SWAP: Mac's refrigerator section has other snack options. A Clover Leaf Tuna Salad Kit, classic flavour, which comes with six crackers, a small can of tuna, a white paper napkin and a baby plastic spoon, has 160 calories, 5 grams of fat and 250 mg of sodium. Its 14 grams of protein will help keep your hunger at bay until the next meal.

7-Eleven: Monterey Jack and Chicken Go-Go Taquitos

Go-Go Taquitos—flour tortillas stuffed with a filling, then battered and deep-fried—are the most popular snacks at 7-Eleven. The kind filled with Monterey Jack cheese and diced chicken is the favourite flavour. Deep-fry anything and it's bound to taste good. But ask yourself, is this really the best thing to be grabbing for a snack? Ten bites will net you 560 calories—one-quarter of what most people should consume in a day. That's too many calories in too few bites. These Go-Go Taquitos will be go-go-gone before you get 560 calories' worth of enjoyment out of them.

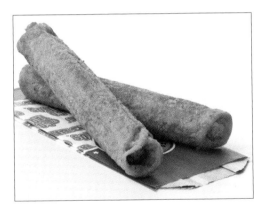

Serving size: 2 Monterey Jack and Chicken Go-Go Taquitos
Calories: 560
Fat: 28 grams
Carbohydrates: 60 grams
Protein: 14 grams
Sodium: 1,560 mg
Salt shakes: 39

SMART SWAP: Walk right past the hot food to the sandwich cooler for one of 7-Eleven's fresh sandwiches, which clock in at under 400 calories. Eat half for a substantial snack.

Shoppers Drug Mart: Smartfood popcorn and chocolate milk

One hundred years ago, it was general stores that supplied a community with all its needs. Now, it's Shoppers Drug Mart.

The warehouse-sized space sells *everything:* medication, bandages, bug spray, hair care products, mascara, diapers, perfume, nail clippers, candles and, most recently, groceries. Snacks, too. Many, many kinds of snacks.

If you're looking for a healthy nibble when shopping for shampoo, you may think a bag of Smartfood popcorn and a 500 mL carton of chocolate milk will do the trick. The snack will provide some fibre, protein and calcium. But finish the bag and drain the carton and you'll have consumed 600 calories and 23 grams of fat—more than twice as many of each as what's in a Harvey's grilled chicken sandwich.

SMART SWAPS: Individual-sized foods have ballooned in recent years. All too often, that snack-sized bag will have at least twice as many calories as you need for a mid-afternoon nibble. It's usually best to split these packages.

If you won't be able to eat just half the bag of Smartfood popcorn, leave it on the shelf. Instead, pick up a box of granola bars—look for a brand made with whole grains and that has at least 4 grams of fibre per bar. Eat one bar and leave the box in your car for the next time you get caught hungry between meals.

It's an easy switch for the chocolate milk. Grab the 250 mL carton. It will satisfy your sweet tooth and your stomach grumbles for 150 fewer calories and just 2.5 grams of fat.

SMARTFOOD POPCORN
Serving size: 55 grams
Calories: 300
Fat: 18 grams
Carbohydrates: 28 grams
   (including 4 grams fibre)
Protein: 7 grams
Sodium: 440 mg
Salt shakes: 11

Best before / Meilleur avant ▶

04 1513 02:49

Neilson.
1% partly
M.F. skimmed
chocolate milk

fresh
1% partly
M.F. skimmed
chocolate
milk
keep refrigerated
500 mL

Shake Well

AN EXCELLENT SOURCE OF CALCIUM

Smartfood

POPCORN

MAÏS
SOUFFLÉ

À SAVEUR DE
FROMAGE
WHITE CHEDDAR BLAN
CHEESE FLAVOURED

FRAÎCHEUR GARANTIE
GUARANTEED FRESH
· UNTIL PRINTED DATE ·
· DATE INDIQUÉE ·

CHOCOLATE MILK
Serving size: 500 mL carton
Calories: 300
Fat: 5 grams
Carbohydrates: 54 grams
   (including 50 grams sugars)
Protein: 14 grams
Sodium: 420 mg
Salt shakes: 10 1/2

Go nuts

Natural, or raw, nuts are one of nature's best snacks. They are packed with protein and filled with nutrients and are a rich source of heart-healthy monounsaturated fat. Plus they are portable, easy to munch on and tasty.

Almonds

Recommended serving size: 1/4 cup, about 25 almonds
Calories: 209

Benefits: The 12 grams of monounsaturated fat found in a single serving of almonds helps to cut LDL (bad) cholesterol and boost HDL (good) cholesterol in your bloodstream. A serving of almonds also provides you with 4 grams of fibre and a dose of magnesium and calcium.

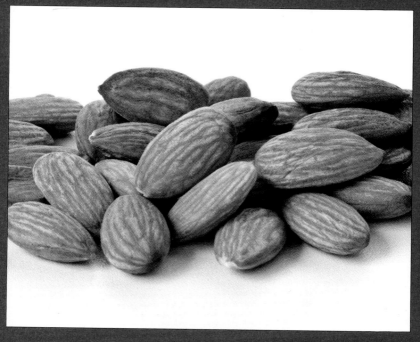

Walnuts

Recommended serving size: 1/4 cup, about 14 walnut halves

Calories: 166

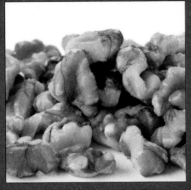

Benefits: Gram for gram, walnuts contain more omega-3 fatty acids than any other kind of nut. Omega-3 fatty acids help protect heart health by preventing blood clots, and research has shown them to lower the risk of chronic diseases, including cancer, heart disease and arthritis. Walnuts are also a source of vitamin B, calcium and magnesium.

Peanuts

Recommended serving size: 1/4 cup, about 30 peanuts,
**   or 2 tablespoons natural peanut butter**

Calories: 217

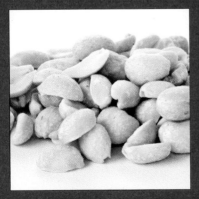

Benefits: Peanuts—a legume, of course, not a nut—pack a wallop of phytosterols, plant compounds that help prevent our bodies from absorbing cholesterol. Research has shown that people who regularly eat peanuts or other nuts are at lower risk of fatal heart attacks. A serving of peanuts also contains 3 grams of fibre and is a source of folate, a water-soluble B vitamin that helps produce and maintain new cells.

Know your nuts

Once they have left the farm, not all nuts are "made" the same. Nuts that have been kettle-cooked, seasoned or honey-roasted could have added fat and will be high in sodium. It's important to investigate labels to find the best-for-you nuts.

While both these packages have roughly the same amount of calories and grams of fat, the natural almonds are the hands-down winner. They have a minuscule amount of sodium compared with the 580 mg in the peanuts. And "natural almonds" are the only ingredient. The pack of peanuts has an ingredient list 11 items long.

Life kettle-cooked peanuts, sea salt and malt vinegar flavour
Serving size: 70 grams
Calories: 450
Fat: 36 grams
Carbohydrates: 14 grams
   (including 8 grams fibre)
Protein: 15 grams
Sodium: 580 mg
Salt shakes: 14 1/2

Life natural almonds
Serving size: 70 grams
Calories: 440
Fat: 36 grams
Carbohydrates: 14 grams
   (including 8 grams fibre)
Protein: 14 grams
Sodium: 5 mg
Salt shakes: < 1

Beware: Both packages are way too big for one snack. A serving of nuts is about 30 grams, not 70. So open the package, pour out a palmful of nuts (about 1/4 cup) and save the remainder for the following day.

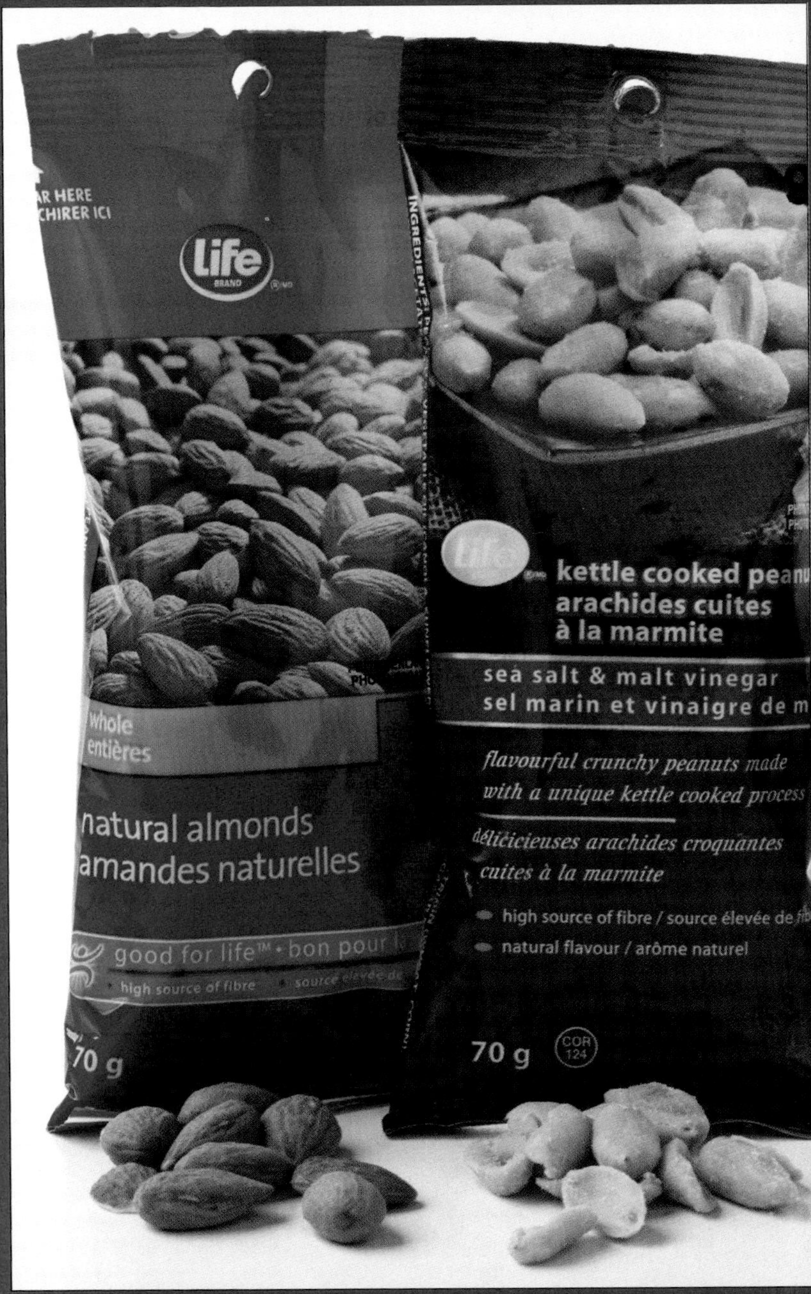

AR HERE
CHIRER ICI
Life
whole
entières
natural almonds
amandes naturelles
good for life™ • bon pour
high source of fibre
70 g
kettle cooked pea
arachides cuites
à la marmite
sea salt & malt vinegar
sel marin et vinaigre de m
flavourful crunchy peanuts made
with a unique kettle cooked process
délicicieuses arachides croquantes
cuites à la marmite
high source of fibre / source élevée de
natural flavour / arôme naturel
70 g
COR
124

Snack and energy bars

Few snacks are handier to eat on the run than prepackaged bars. Between granola bars, protein bars, nut bars and energy bars, there are a dizzying number of choices in the snack aisles. Some are healthy. Many are loaded with sugar, making them more like candy bars than nutritious snacks.

Kellogg's Vector Energy Bar, chocolate-chip flavour

The calories, fat and protein in this bar ensure it will be satisfying. But for mild hunger pangs, it has too many calories. Grab this only when you know your next meal is a long way off.

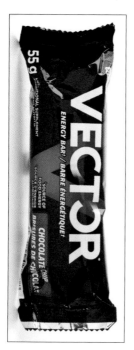

Serving size: 55 grams

Calories: 230

Fat: 7 grams

Carbohydrates: 32 grams (sugars not provided;
    2.5 grams fibre)

Protein: 9 grams

Sodium: 85 mg

Salt shakes: 2

Kashi TLC Fruit & Grain Bar, pumpkin pie flavour

This Kashi Fruit & Grain bar provides 4 grams of beneficial fibre for just 130 calories. And you get seven different whole grains—something Canadians don't get enough of. Pair this bar with a piece of fruit and you have a standout snack.

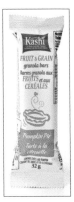

Serving size: 32 grams

Calories: 130

Fat: 3 grams

Carbohydrates: 21 grams (including 8 grams sugars; 4 grams fibre)

Protein: 4 grams

Sodium: 45 mg

Salt shakes: 1

Life Granola Bar, mixed berries and nuts flavour

The 4 grams of fibre for 140 calories makes this bar a standout too. Plus it has no artificial flavours, colours or preservatives.

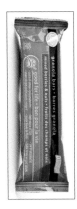

Serving size: 35 grams

Calories: 140

Fat: 3.5 grams

Carbohydrates: 25 grams (including 9 grams sugars; 4 grams fibre)

Protein: 3 grams

Sodium: 45 mg

Salt shakes: 1

Clif Bar, crunchy peanut butter flavour

This Clif Bar's 250 calories and 12 grams of protein will keep an active athlete powering through an afternoon ride through the mountains. For less active folks, Clif has too much heft for a simple snack. This is one that should be split, either with a friend or with yourself over the day.

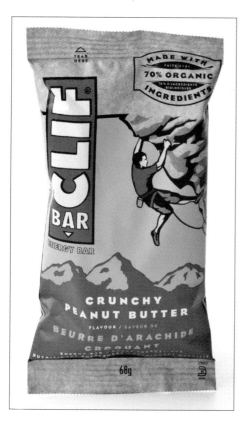

Serving size: 68 grams

Calories: 250

Fat: 6 grams

Carbohydrates: 40 grams
(including 18 grams sugars;
4 grams fibre)

Protein: 12 grams

Sodium: 250 mg

Salt shakes: 6

Quaker Chewy Granola Bar, chocolate-chip flavour

At first glance, this bar's nutrition numbers look the best of the lot. But size-wise, Quaker weighs between 6 and 42 grams less than the other bars. Make its serving size match the others and this chocolate-chip bar—really, more like a chewy oatmeal cookie—has as many calories as its neighbours.

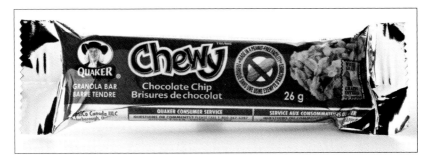

Serving size: 26 grams

Calories: 110

Fat: 3 grams

Carbohydrates: 19 grams (including 5 grams sugars; 2 grams fibre)

Protein: 1 gram

Sodium: 60 mg

Salt shakes: 1 1/2

HOW TO SPOT A NUTRITIOUS BAR: Scan the nutrition label and list of ingredients and check the serving size. Granola bars vary widely in size. Pick ones that list whole grains, such as oats, as the first ingredient, have 4 or more grams of fibre, less than 10 grams of sugar and no trans fat.

Tim Hortons apple fritter

A doughnut might be the iconic Canadian snack. Calorie-wise, an apple should take the crown and the fruit is as much a Canuck as a Timmies doughnut. But never, ever will we give up our doughnuts.

Sweetened dough fried in oil and topped—in some cases also filled—with sugar will never win any health awards. But if this is an occasional treat, a doughnut can't do too much dietary damage.

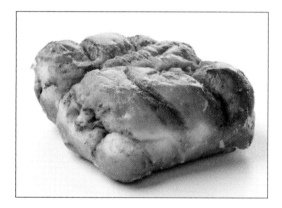

Calories: 300
Fat: 11 grams
Carbohydrates: 49
    grams (including 16
    grams sugars; 2
    grams fibre)
Protein: 4 grams
Sodium: 350 mg
Salt shakes: 9

FAST FACT: At Tim Hortons, the calorie count of different doughnuts is rarely the same. With 360 calories and 23 grams of fat, the walnut crunch is the worst of the bakery's bunch. Maple, chocolate or honey-dipped doughnuts are on the other side of the spectrum with 210 calories and 8 grams of fat.

DOUGHNUT DILEMMA

1 honey cruller

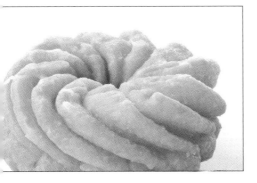

Calories: 320
Fat: 19 grams
Carbohydrates: 37 grams
   (including 23 grams sugars;
   0 grams fibre)
Protein: 1 gram
Sodium: 220 mg
Salt shakes: 5 1/2

HAS MORE CALORIES THAN

3 Timbits

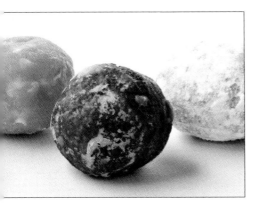

SMART SWAP: Get three Timbits instead of a single doughnut. All together, a honey-dipped, chocolate-glazed and strawberry-filled Timbit will net you 190 calories and 6.5 grams of fat. You get three different doughnuts *and* save 130 calories and 12.5 grams of fat!

Ikea cinnamon bun

Most people don't go to Ikea for a snack. They go for couches, kitchens or architecturally interesting vases. But it sure is hard to sneak past the Exit Cafe without nipping in for a warm, sweet-scented cinnamon bun.

Ikea's cinnamon buns aren't the biggest—they're about the size of the palm of your hand. And the snack, in comparison to other on-the-go treats, is fairly reasonable with 276 calories and 6 grams of fat. But the calories, which come from processed and refined carbohydrates—including a lot of sugar—aren't satiating and will leave snackers hungry soon after eating the bun.

Calories: 276
Fat: 6 grams
Carbohydrates: 50 grams
Protein: 5 grams
Sodium: 147 mg
Salt shakes: 3 1/2

SMART SWAPS: You could split the bun to share with your shopping companion over a cup of coffee. You could opt for a cone of frozen yogurt for 118 calories and about 2 grams of fat. Or, you could walk right past Ikea's Exit Cafe, content with the new pretty pillow tucked into your shopping bag.

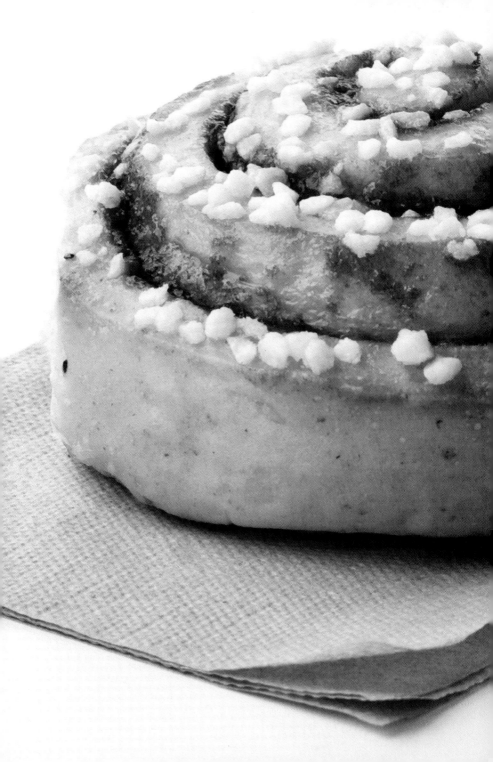

McDonald's Grilled Chicken Snack Wrap

McDonald's is known for its supersize meals. But in recent years, snack-sized sandwiches, wraps and icy treats have started to take over the menu. The fast food king should be given kudos for offering smaller options that are as quick and convenient as the much-maligned Big Mac. But in the calorie department, these "snacks" are often more like mini-meals.

Calories: 230
Fat: 8 grams
Carbohydrates: 24 grams (including 3 grams fibre)
Protein: 16 grams
Sodium: 490 mg
Salt shakes: 12

SMART SWAP: McDonald's Fruit 'n Yogurt Parfait is a true snack. It has 180 calories, 2 grams of fat and just 100 mg of sodium. Its 6 grams of protein will help chase away hunger.

MEGAN'S TIP: A dietitian friend once recommended forgoing the Snack Wrap's creamy sauce to cut calories and fat. I love this tip! Now, I always order my Snack Wrap without sauce and hardly notice a difference in taste.

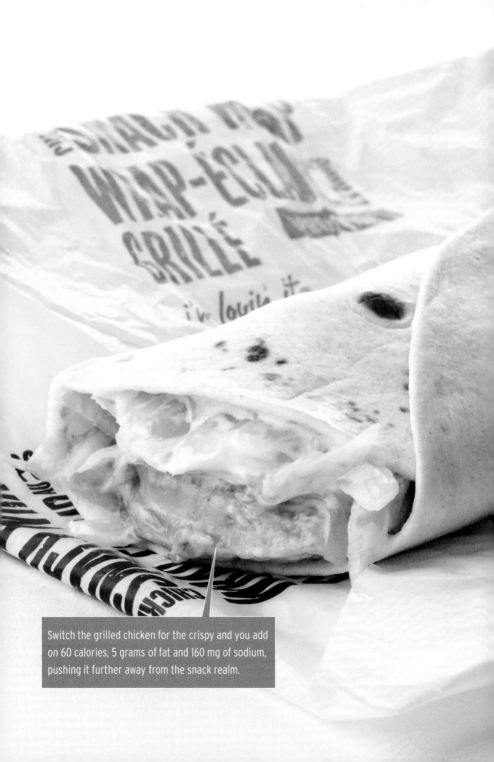

Switch the grilled chicken for the crispy and you add on 60 calories, 5 grams of fat and 160 mg of sodium, pushing it further away from the snack realm.

Super satisfying snacks

Whether you're at the gas station, corner store or coffee shop, spend a few more minutes scouting for snacks and you'll likely find one of these nutritious choices. Better yet, keep a selection of healthy snacks on hand. Maybe tuck a few into your desk drawer or keep your fridge stocked with healthful alternatives to the fast-food world's versions of snacks.

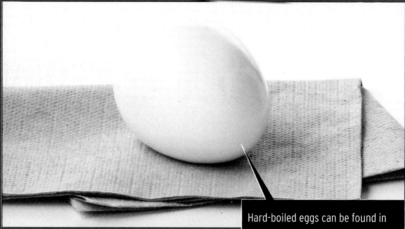

Hard-boiled eggs can be found in some supermarkets and convenience stores. They are sold as a pair, already peeled and protected in sealed plastic.

Hard-boiled egg

Calories: 70

Fat: 5 grams

Carbohydrates: 1 gram

Protein: 6 grams

Sodium: 63 mg

Salt shakes: 1 1/2

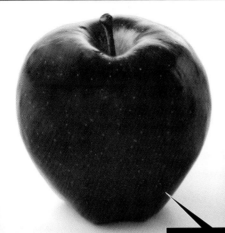

Apple
Calories: 110
Fat: 0 grams
Carbohydrates: 29 grams
  (including 4 grams fibre)
Protein: 0.5 grams
Sodium: 2 mg
Salt shakes: 0

Eat apple slices with 1 tablespoon of natural peanut butter for an additional 4 grams of hunger-busting protein and just 92 additional calories.

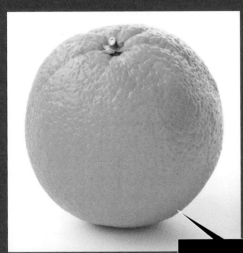

Orange
Calories: 86
Fat: 0 grams
Carbohydrates: 21 grams
  (including 3 grams fibre)
Protein: 1 gram
Sodium: 0 mg
Salt shakes: 0

A serving of just about any fruit or vegetable will make a fantastic snack.

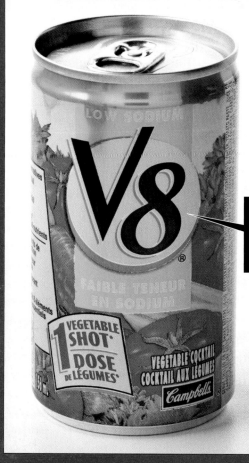

Regular V8 is awash in sodium. If you like veggie juice, make sure you sip the low-sodium version.

Low-sodium V8 vegetable cocktail

Serving size: 156 mL can

Calories: 35

Carbohydrates: 7 grams
   (including 5 grams sugars;
   2 grams fibre)

Fat: 0 grams

Protein: 1 gram

Sodium: 85 mg

Salt shakes: 2

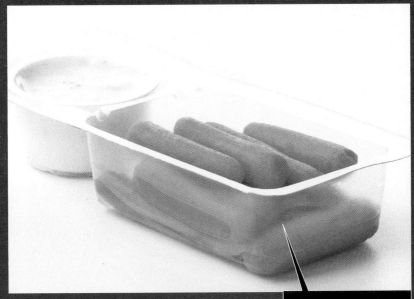

Sobeys baby carrots with dip

Calories: 70

Fat: 5 grams

Carbohydrates: 6 grams
   (including 4 grams sugars; 1 gram fibre)

Protein: 1 gram

Sodium: 210 mg

Salt shakes: 5

Swap out the carrots for any variety of vegetable. Keep a selection of green beans, mini-cucumbers, cherry tomatoes and snow peas washed and ready to go in the fridge.

Mini Babybel cheese

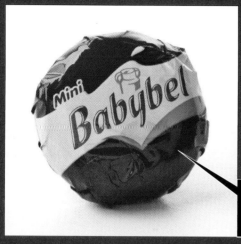

Serving size: 20 grams
Calories: 60
Fat: 5 grams
Carbohydrates: 0 grams
Protein: 4 grams
Sodium: 135 mg
Salt shakes: 3

A single serving of cottage cheese or low-fat yogurt would be just as ideal as this tiny wheel of cheese.

Summer Fresh Snack'n Go hummus and flatbread pack

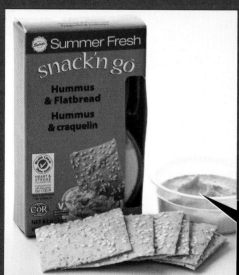

Calories: 170
Fat: 9 grams
Carbohydrates: 24 grams
   (including 2 grams
   sugars; 3 grams fibre)
Protein: 6 grams
Sodium: 280 mg
Salt shakes: 7

If you have a food processor, making a batch of hummus with canned beans is a breeze—and you can control the fat and sodium levels.

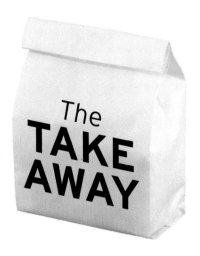

The
TAKE
AWAY

Snack strategically. Give your snack selecting as much attention as you do your meal choosing.

Watch out for snacks that are more like mini-meals. The ideal snack has 200 calories or less.

Pick snacks that have spent as little time in a factory as possible. Minimally processed foods—think fruit, nuts, yogurt, vegetables—offer so much more nutritionally than ones sealed in packages and sitting on a shelf. And they are likely to have fewer calories.

Plan ahead so you're not caught on the highway with only convenience stores as your hunger respite. Most snacks from home can be easily stashed in a bag. Keep a lunch cooler in the car and pack an extra egg or a cup of yogurt to eat on the way home.

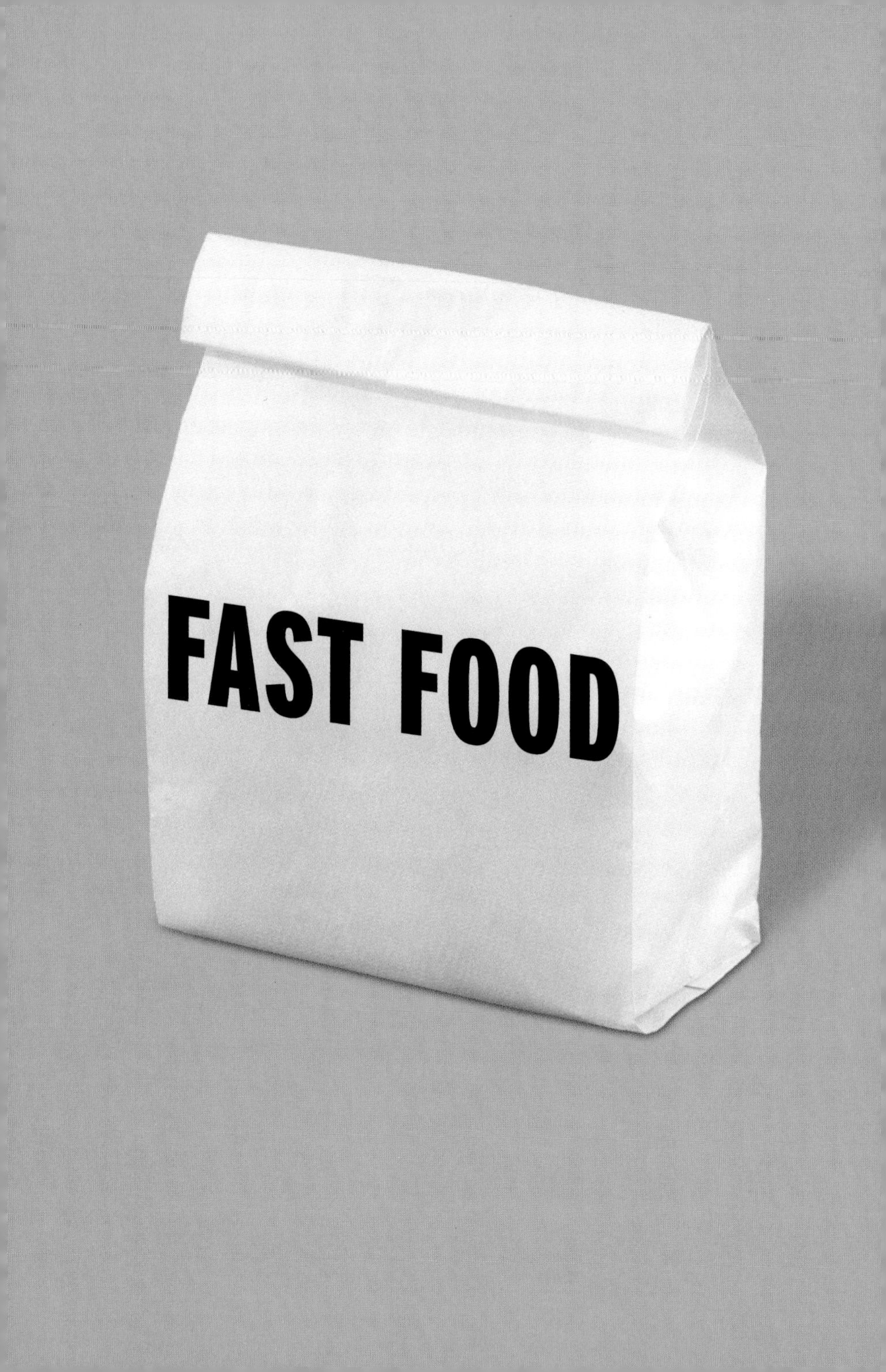
FAST FOOD

One of the best things about fast food is that you can get it, well, fast.

Some days, grabbing a meal in mere minutes after dashing in off the sidewalk or zooming through the drive-thru is the only way to fit food into a schedule. On those craziest of days, a craving can easily overcome common sense. But take a few extra seconds, and a few calming breaths, and you can make a fast-food choice that will satisfy a craving and keep calories in check.

>

Burgers

A patty of ground beef, set inside a fluffy white bun. Burgers can be simple affairs. But in the 50 years since first becoming a fast-food staple, burgers have ballooned into behemoths. These days, the traditional, one-patty burger is often ranked lowest on fast-food menus. The ones made with two patties, double cheese, sautéed mushrooms, bacon and deep-fried onions get all the attention. Even the Big Mac—the once infamous double-patty creation—is relatively tame with its 540 calories. Modern mega-calorie burgers clock in with double the damage.

If you're starting to roll your eyes, that's fine. Some of us will always believe the bigger the burger, the better. For others who would rather not down 800 calories in a single sandwich, it is possible to order a sensible burger at the fast-food counter.

Tips for a better burger

- Skip the cheese. You'll save between 50 and 80 calories and about 5 grams of fat. With everything else going on inside the bun, you won't even miss the taste.
- Ditto with the creamy sauces. A tablespoon of mayonnaise, for example, has about 100 calories and 11 grams of fat.
- Ignore burgers described as ultimate, deluxe or supreme. Burgers labelled with these kinds of adjectives will typically have at least 300 more calories and double the fat of a plain ole burger.

Megan's Tip: Most fast-food joints offer smaller versions of their flagship burger. They may look tiny compared with their big-boy cousins. But the junior burgers are closer—in size and in calories—to what you should be eating for a meal. After looking at the nutrition numbers, I've decided to satisfy my burger cravings for under 300 calories by ordering junior-sized fast-food.

Burgers at a glance

Burger	Calories	Fat (g)	Sodium (mg)	Salt shakes
A&W Grandpa Burger with cheese	810	50	1,550	39
A&W Mama Burger	400	19	850	21
Burger King Triple Whopper with cheese	1,250	84	1,600	40
Burger King Whopper Jr	340	19	610	15
Harvey's Original Hamburger	380	16	980	24 1/2
McDonald's Angus Burger with bacon and cheese	780	44	1,990	50
McDonald's Hamburger	250	8	510	13
Wendy's Baconator Double Hamburger	980	64	1,960	49
Wendy's 1/4 lb Single Hamburger	590	33	1,170	29

Harvey's Original Hamburger

Harvey's says it'll make your hamburger a beautiful thing. You should take it up on the offer and build a burger that's big on taste but lower in calories. Harvey's gives you a strong head start, since its original burger is lower in calories and fat than almost any other fast-food burger of comparable size.

Without garnishes
Calories: 380
Fat: 16 grams
Carbohydrates: 37 grams
Protein: 20 grams
Sodium: 980 mg
Salt shakes: 24

DANGER ZONE: Watch out for the extras. Harvey's spicy mesquite sauce will add 140 calories and 14 grams of fat to your burger.

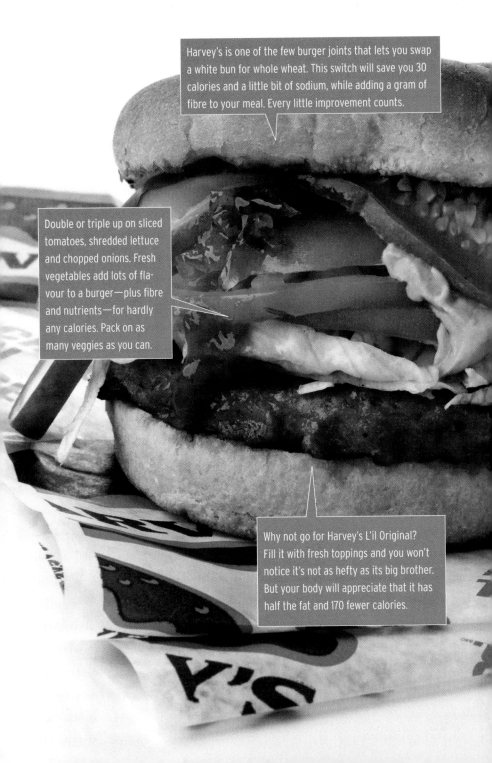

Harvey's is one of the few burger joints that lets you swap a white bun for whole wheat. This switch will save you 30 calories and a little bit of sodium, while adding a gram of fibre to your meal. Every little improvement counts.

Double or triple up on sliced tomatoes, shredded lettuce and chopped onions. Fresh vegetables add lots of flavour to a burger—plus fibre and nutrients—for hardly any calories. Pack on as many veggies as you can.

Why not go for Harvey's L'il Original? Fill it with fresh toppings and you won't notice it's not as hefty as its big brother. But your body will appreciate that it has half the fat and 170 fewer calories.

Chicken sandwiches

It's a common misconception that a chicken burger is better for you than one made with beef. At home, where you are in control of cooking the bird, that may be the case. But in the fast-food world, chicken burgers do not get top marks for health. They will often have as many calories as standard beef burgers. The obligatory mayo topping adds plenty of fat. And the seasoned chicken is saturated with salt, bestowing many chicken burgers with as much sodium as your body needs in a day. You'll need to pick wisely and make a few simple swaps for a chicken burger to get back its health halo.

Tips for a better chicken sandwich

- Grilled chicken is, of course, a better choice than crispy. Opt for chicken that hasn't gone into the deep fryer will save between 100 and 150 calories and between 10 and 20 grams of fat.
- Mayo is the condiment of choice on chicken sandwiches. But try leaving it off your next order; you likely won't miss it, since the chicken itself has so much seasoning. At Burger King, for example, ditching the mayo on the Original Chicken Sandwich will save you 23 grams of fat—more than the amount in a medium order of BK onion rings.
- Consider ordering the junior version of a chicken sandwich. Downsizing will save you at least 100 calories and 10 grams of fat.

Chicken sandwiches at a glance

Sandwich	Calories	Fat (g)	Sodium (mg)	Salt shakes
A&W Chubby Chicken Burger	480	26	1,230	31
Burger King Original Chicken Sandwich	680	43	1,430	36
Burger King Tendergrill	370	16	910	23
Harvey's Crispy Chicken	470	16	1,320	33
Harvey's Grilled Chicken	290	5	810	20
McDonald's McChicken Sandwich	490	27	790	20
McDonald's McBistro Southwest Crispy Chicken	560	28	1,020	25 1/2
Wendy's Spicy Chicken Breast Sandwich	510	21	1,240	31
Wendy's Ultimate Chicken Grill	380	10	1,010	25

A&W Chubby Chicken Burger

One wonders why A&W called its chicken sandwich chubby. Promising plumpness isn't usually a selling point for diners.

If you're looking for something leaner, a few modifications can take the chubby out of this chicken burger.

Calories: 480
Fat: 26 grams
Carbohydrates: 44 grams
Protein: 21 grams
Sodium: 1,230 mg
Salt shakes: 31

DANGER ZONE: Don't undo those smart swaps by ordering A&W's root beer milkshake. This signature concoction contains 700 calories and 18 grams of fat and has the equivalent of 25 cubes of sugar. For the *regular* size!

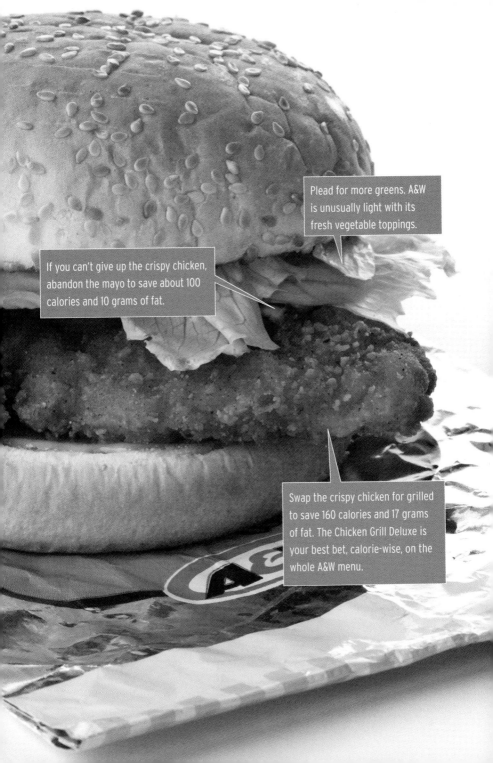

Condiments count

With all the calories and fat hiding in fast food, sodium may not be your top concern. But consider this: pile on too many condiments and you'll have topped your burger with one-half of your day's worth of sodium.

Once I found out about all the sodium lurking in garnishes, I started topping my burgers with a judicious smear of my favourite condiment—spicy mustard—and layers of fresh vegetables. I usually ask for triple tomatoes.

Dare to Compare: Just 1 tablespoon each of ketchup, mustard and relish, plus two pickle slices, has 593 mg of sodium, about the same amount as what's in 114 corn chips.

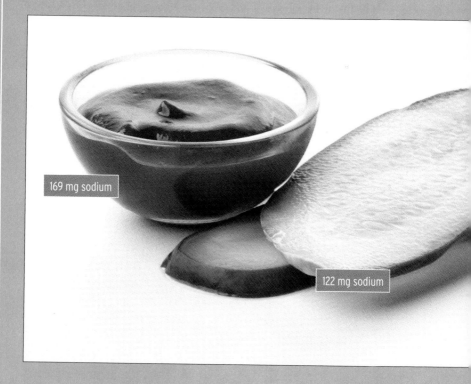

169 mg sodium

122 mg sodium

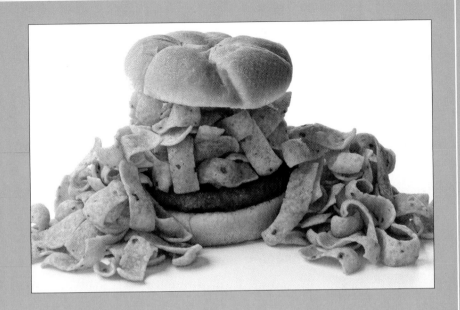

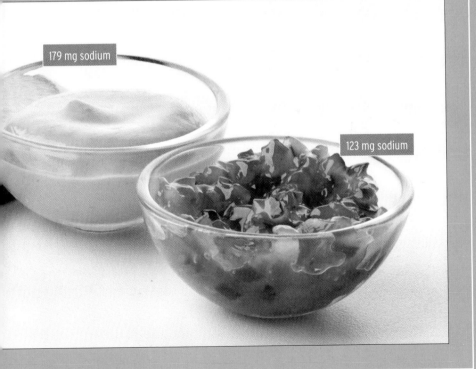

179 mg sodium

123 mg sodium

Is it better to go veggie?

If you're a vegetarian, the answer to that question is a simple and emphatic *yes*. But for those who think a veggie burger is a lighter option than one made with meat, the answer is not so simple.

Some patties are deep-fried, just like a chicken burger. Others are pan-fried in oil. Many are filled with a long list of ingredients to make them taste succulent and beefy. Almost all are highly seasoned, and some can pack as much sodium as a bacon-topped beef burger. Bottom line? Few fast-food veggie burgers deserve a health halo.

If you are strictly concerned with calories, it may be best to order the smallest version of a beef burger and garnish wisely.

If you are trying to limit your intake of red meat, a veggie burger can satisfy a beef burger craving. But it's probably best to inquire about the ingredient list. Some veggie burgers contain trans fat or are made of highly processed ingredients that bear no resemblance to vegetables.

Vegetarian burgers at a glance

Burger	Calories	Fat (g)	Sodium (mg)	Salt shakes
A&W Veggie Deluxe	410	17	1,340	33 1/2
Burger King veggie burger	270	6	640	16
Harvey's veggie burger	290	10	580	14 1/2
KFC veggie burger	440	19	980	24 1/2

Do you want fries with that?

We consider fries the side that goes with a sandwich. But unlike a slice of pickle, a medium order of fries can pack hundreds of calories and up to a third of your day's worth of fat. It's pretty much like eating an extra burger with your burger.

Whose fries are the best bet? If you consider just the calories and fat, the fries at these fast-food giants are pretty much the same. The small differences are primarily due to portion size. If you look at sodium, McDonald's wins the fight—even if you order its fries with salt—and Harvey's sinks to the bottom of the list.

Fries at a glance

Fries (medium/regular)	Calories	Fat (g)	Sodium (mg)	Salt shakes
A&W (135 grams)	410	17	730	18
Burger King (116 grams)	350	17	790	20
Harvey's (120 grams)	320	13	950	24
McDonald's (113 grams)	360	17	270	7
Wendy's (142 grams)	420	20	470	12

French fry facts

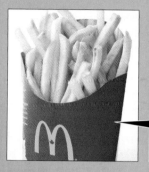

McDonald's french fries
Ask for your fries unsalted and the sodium count will drop to an impressive 50 mg.

> More fat and calories than a McDonald's cheeseburger with bacon.

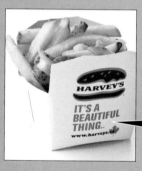

Harvey's french fries
Why not get the value size? It will satisfy your hankering for fries for 190 calories and 7 grams of fat.

> The same amount of fat and calories as a Harvey's hot dog.

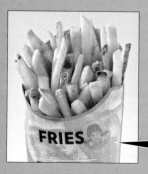

Wendy's french fries
Consider swapping the fries for a baked potato with sour cream and chives. This hearty side has 360 calories, 6 grams of fat and 75 mg of sodium. Plus a whole lot more nutrients than fries.

> More fat and calories than Wendy's Homestyle Chicken Strips.

Burger King french fries

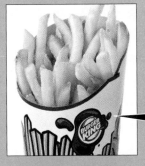

Like McDonald's, Burger King will make fries un-salted. But this omission will save only 140 mg of sodium.

More fat and calories than BK's cheese-burger.

A&W french fries

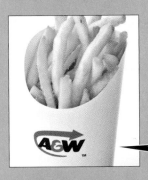

Dunk your fries in gravy, and you add 100 calories, 6 grams of fat and a stunning 730 mg of sodium—filing this side with as much sodium as your body needs in a day.

About the same calories and fat as four Chubby Chicken Strips.

A Losing Proposition: If you eat a regular order of fries three times a week, you add between 1,000 and 1,200 calories to your diet. Cut out just one weekly order and you could lose 6 pounds over the course of a year.

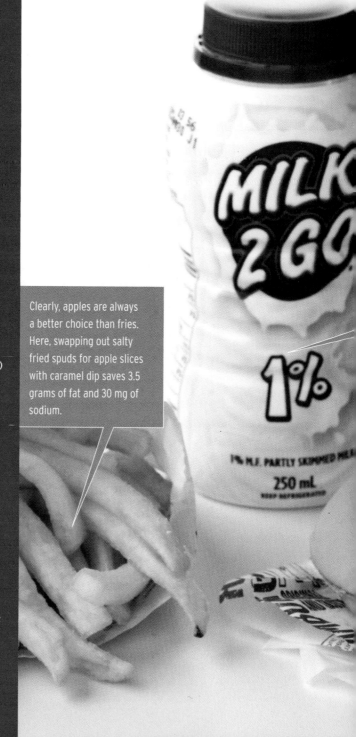

HAMBURGER
Calories: 250
Fat: 8 grams
Carbohydrates: 32 grams
(including 7 grams sugars;
2 grams fibre)
Protein: 12 grams
Sodium: 510 mg
Salt shakes: 13

MINI FRY
Calories: 100
Fat: 4.5 grams
Carbohydrates: 13 grams
(including 1 gram fibre)
Protein: 1 gram
Sodium: 70 mg
Salt shakes: 2

MILK
Serving size: 250 mL
Calories: 110
Fat: 2.5 grams
Carbohydrates: 12 grams
(including 12 grams sugars)
Protein: 9 grams
Sodium: 120 mg
Salt shakes: 3

STRAWBERRY DANINO
YOGURT
Calories: 45
Fat: 0.5 grams
Carbohydrates: 6 grams
(including 5 grams sugars)
Protein: 2 grams
Sodium: 25 mg
Salt shakes: 0.5

TOTAL
Calories: 505
Fat: 15.5 grams
Carbohydrates: 76 grams
(including 21 grams sugars;
4 grams fibre)
Protein: 23 grams
Sodium: 870 mg
Salt shakes: 22

Clearly, apples are always
a better choice than fries.
Here, swapping out salty
fried spuds for apple slices
with caramel dip saves 3.5
grams of fat and 30 mg of
sodium.

McDonald's Happy Meal

It's the iconic kids' meal, the one that every child wants. Sometimes desire for a Happy Meal is fuelled by the tricked-out cardboard container or a ketchup-y burger. Most times, it's fuelled by the toy. The good news is that its mix-and-match menu can be a reasonable, once-in-a-while treat—if you choose the right items.

Health Canada recommends children between the ages of four and nine get two to three servings of dairy products each day, yet about one-third of kids don't meet that daily requirement. Why order a pop when milk has so many benefits?

Okay, so your kid won't get the toy and that might be a deal-breaker. But if you are hitting the drive-thru for a quick dinner before soccer practice, and nutrition trumps the need for a toy, consider ordering your child a chicken fajita with a Fruit 'n Yogurt Parfait. This pairing (with a bottle of water) has a total of 380 calories, 7.5 grams of fat and 565 mg of sodium.

This is one of the Happy Meal's better main courses, despite its saltiness. The cheeseburger has 50 more calories and 4 more grams of fat, while the four-piece Chicken McNuggets with sweet and sour sauce have 4 more grams of fat and 30 mg more sodium.

Pizza

In elementary school we were taught that pizza is the ideal dish because it's made with ingredients from each of the four food groups. This nutrition advice still holds true—but with some parameters. The pizza crust can't be pillow-thick, or stuffed with cheese. The mozzarella can't be spread on by the handful. A pizza can't mimic a cheeseburger or Buffalo chicken wings. And creamy dips should definitely not come on the side.

A pizza can be a diet in a box, if you order right. But it can just as easily be a diet buster.

Tips for a better pizza

- Choose thin-crust over hand-tossed, regular or deep-dish dough. A thin crust on a medium pizza will save between 300 and 400 calories at Domino's, Little Caesars and Pizza Hut.
- Stick with traditional marinara sauce (maybe even double it). You'll get a dose of vegetables and it will always be the lowest calorie option.
- Ask for your pizza to be made with half the usual amount of cheese. A light layer will still give that gooey taste and will save between 150 and 200 calories on a medium pizza. It will also eliminate about 10 grams of fat and 500 mg of sodium.
- Load up on fresh vegetables. Pizza parlours have a wide selection of veggies, from sliced mushrooms to chopped tomatoes to roasted red peppers. There should be one, two or (hopefully) three that you like. These low-cal, nutrient-rich toppings are the best way to build a pizza.
- Beware of salty toppings. Cured meat, pickled peppers, olives and extra cheese will send your pizza's sodium level skyrocketing. On a medium pizza, three of these toppings can add up to 3,000 mg of sodium.

Pizza slices at a glance

Pizza (1 slice)	Calories	Fat (g)	Sodium (mg)	Salt shakes
Domino's, large deep-dish with pizza sauce, extra cheese, pepperoni, mushrooms and green peppers	368	17	887	22
Domino's, large thin-crust with pizza sauce, regular cheese, pineapple and ham	218	10	474	12
Pizza Hut Meat Lover's Stuffed Crust, large	480	22	760	19
Pizza Hut Veggie Lover's Thin 'n Crispy, large	190	6	370	9
Pizza Pizza pepperoni, walk-in slice	630	21	1,600	40

Pizza Pizza pepperoni pizza

A walk-in slice of pepperoni pizza may be one of the easiest fast foods to eat on the go. But you'll have to do a lot of walking to get rid of the calories crammed into this piece of pizza pie. Spend an extra 10 minutes to custom order a small pizza made with a thin crust, half the cheese and more veggies and you can eat four slices of the made-to-order pizza and be better off.

WALK-IN SLICE

Calories: 630

Fat: 21 grams

Carbohydrates: 85 grams

Protein: 32 grams

Sodium: 1,600 mg

Salt shakes: 40

DANGER ZONE: Walk out of Pizza Pizza with a slice of its Bacon Chicken Mushroom Melt Pizza and you'll be eating half your daily calories, half your fat and all of the sodium your body needs in a day.

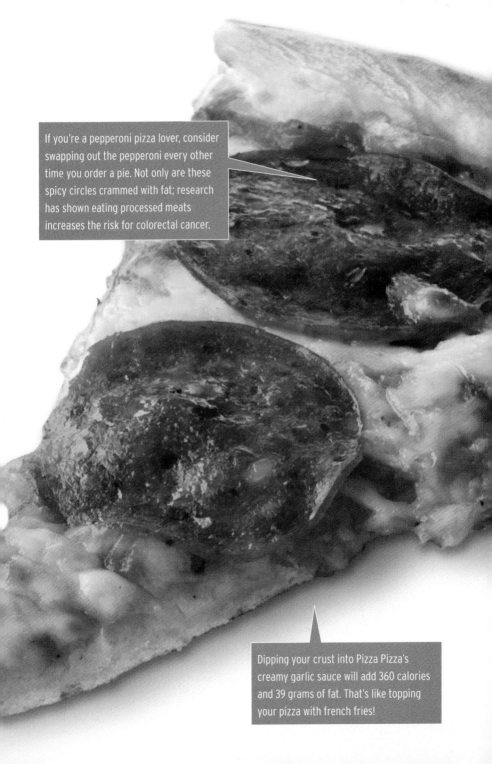

If you're a pepperoni pizza lover, consider swapping out the pepperoni every other time you order a pie. Not only are these spicy circles crammed with fat; research has shown eating processed meats increases the risk for colorectal cancer.

Dipping your crust into Pizza Pizza's creamy garlic sauce will add 360 calories and 39 grams of fat. That's like topping your pizza with french fries!

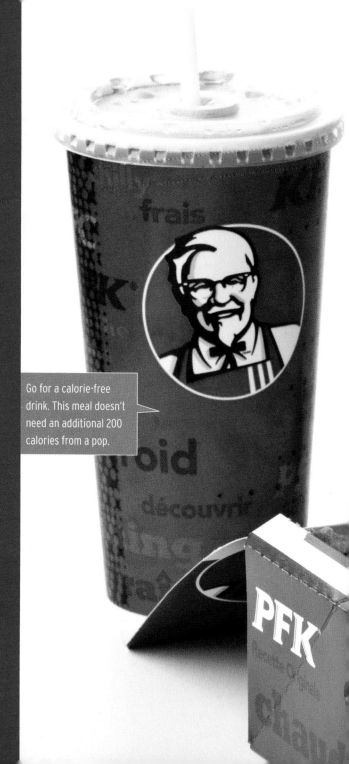

CHICKEN, 1 DRUMSTICK AND 1 KEEL
Calories: 420
Fat: 22 grams
Carbohydrates: 11 grams
Protein: 47 grams
Sodium: 635 mg
Salt shakes: 16

FRENCH FRIES
Calories: 340
Fat: 17 grams
Carbohydrates: 44 grams
Protein: 3 grams
Sodium: 770 mg
Salt shakes: 19

COLESLAW
Calories: 150
Fat: 8 grams
Carbohydrates: 20 grams
Protein: 1 gram
Sodium: 240 mg
Salt shakes: 6

PEPSI, 571 ML
Calories: 241
Carbohydrates: 64 grams

TOTAL
Calories: 1,151
Fat: 47 grams
Carbohydrates: 139 grams
Protein: 51 grams
Sodium: 1,645 mg
Salt shakes: 41

Go for a calorie-free drink. This meal doesn't need an additional 200 calories from a pop.

KFC Two-Piece Meal

Over the years, KFC has tried very hard to make us forget that the *F* in its name stands for "fried." Look at the menu: any reference to a deep fryer has been removed. There's Original Recipe chicken. Hot & Spicy chicken. Crispy chicken. And Popcorn chicken. Despite the clever word tango, all of these chicken pieces have indeed been breaded and fried in oil.

Get the mashed spuds instead and save 260 calories and all the fat.

Consider ordering the crispy chicken strips instead of the chicken pieces. This swap will save you about 100 calories and 7 grams of fat.

Keep this salad. It's the best of the bunch.

What makes a nutritious soup?

Research has shown that soup is especially satiating. Look for soups that contain lots of vegetables, beans or lentils. These chunky versions will help fill you up without filling you out.

Beware creamy soups. Some get their velvety texture from puréed vegetables. Others from a generous glug of cream. It's best to ask about the ingredients before sipping these kinds of soups. For example, at Mr.Sub, a serving of cream of potato and leek soup has 190 calories and 9 grams of fat, while the creamy tomato and roasted red pepper soup has 110 calories and 2.5 grams of fat.

Investigate nutrition numbers to find the least salty soup. They may be hard to track down, but the ideal soups, sodium-wise, are ones that have fewer than 480 mg of sodium per 250 mL.

Soups can be a great way to get more fibre in your day. Look for ones that have at least 2 grams of fibre per 250 mL serving.

Tim Hortons minestrone soup

For the most part, slurping soup will net you a lower calorie lunch. But the big problem with these savoury bowls is their stunning levels of sodium. Just about every restaurant soup—and the ones you get in a can, for that matter—has been liberally laced with salt. Finding one with reasonable seasoning takes a real sodium sleuth.

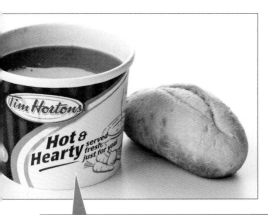

Serving size: 295 mL
Calories: 120
Fat: 1 gram
Carbohydrates: 25 grams
    (including 3 grams fibre)
Protein: 4 grams
Sodium: 660 mg
Salt shakes: 16 1/2

This sensible-sized bowl of soup has more than a third of the sodium your body needs in a day. Do not reach for the paper pack of salt. It needs no other seasoning.

DANGER ZONE: A piece of garlic toast will set you back only 170 calories. But the small piece of bread adds 8 grams of fat and 320 mg of sodium to your meal. The homestyle mini-bun is the better choice.

McDonald's Mighty Caesar Entrée Salad with warm grilled chicken

For the most part, fast-food salads offer more, nutritionally, than the standard burger fare. Still, you will need to choose carefully from the salad offerings. A creamy dressing, some crispy chicken or crunchy bits of bacon and other tidbits can quickly turn a salad into the calorie equal of a greasy burger.

Calories: 610

Fat: 46 grams

Carbohydrates: 17 grams (including 3 grams fibre)

Protein: 27 grams

Sodium: 1,130 mg

Salt shakes: 28

DANGER ZONE: Get crispy chicken on your Mighty Caesar and squirt on a full pack of dressing and your "healthy" salad will clock in with 710 calories, 54 grams of fat and 1,240 mg of sodium. That's like downing McDonald's Double Quarter Pounder with cheese. Seriously.

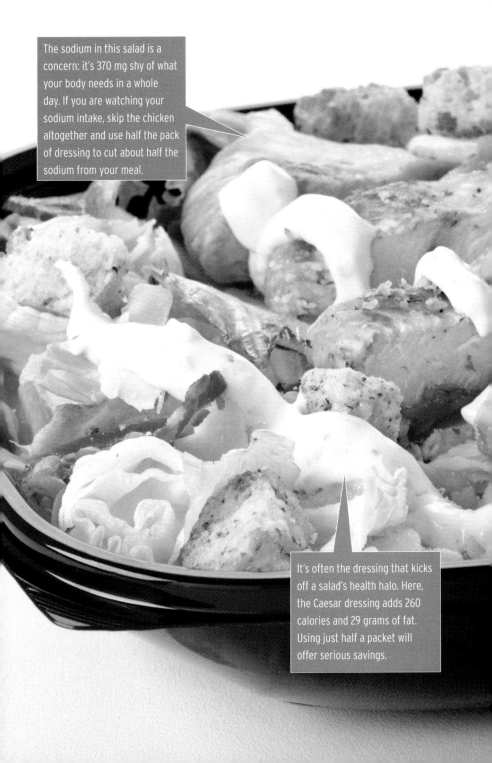

The sodium in this salad is a concern: it's 370 mg shy of what your body needs in a whole day. If you are watching your sodium intake, skip the chicken altogether and use half the pack of dressing to cut about half the sodium from your meal.

It's often the dressing that kicks off a salad's health halo. Here, the Caesar dressing adds 260 calories and 29 grams of fat. Using just half a packet will offer serious savings.

Sandwiches

Some days, nothing satisfies like a sandwich. But like every food, some sandwiches are better for you than others. And just one or two ingredients can be the difference between a sandwich that's nutritious and one that's disastrous to your health.

Tips for a better sandwich

- Choose bread made with whole grains, the more grains the better. This is a great chance in your day to boost your intake of whole grains and fibre.
- Most sandwiches are made with deli meats. But processed meat is one of the foods cancer experts suggest that we limit—or avoid altogether—to reduce the risk of bowel cancer. Look for sandwich shops that offer unprocessed meats.
- Watch out for tuna, egg and seafood salad fillings. These seemingly healthy sandwich stuffings can be extraordinarily high in calories and fat. The tuna salad meant for a 6-inch sub at Subway, for example, has 21 grams of fat—that's about the same amount found in McDonald's Filet-O-Fish sandwich.
- Just as you might for a burger, consider skipping processed cheese on your sandwich. These meagre slices won't add a lot of flavour, but they will add some fat and a lot of sodium.
- Choose condiments wisely. Some sandwich shops offer more than 10 kinds of sauces. At the Pita Pit, a tablespoon of horseradish Dijon has 6 grams of fat and 115 mg of sodium; that's a lot for a small squirt.

Sandwiches at a glance

Sandwich	Calories	Fat (g)	Sodium (mg)	Salt shakes
Mr.Sub grilled chicken sub with lettuce and tomatoes, small size	260	5	560	14
Mr.Sub meatball sub with lettuce, tomatoes and meatball sauce, small size	375	15	930	23
Subway 6-inch turkey sandwich	280	3	790	20
Tim Hortons ham and Swiss sandwich, regular size	380	11	1,200	30
Tim Hortons toasted chicken club sandwich, regular size	370	7	900	22 1/2

Subway 6-inch turkey sandwich

This may be the classic good-for-you sandwich that comes to mind when you imagine a healthy lunch: turkey deli meat, whole-grain bread, lettuce, tomato. If you aren't worried about eating processed meats, then turkey is your best bet for straight-up calorie counting at Subway. The spicy Italian sandwich, however, is one of the poorer choices with 480 calories, 24 grams of fat and 1,520 mg of sodium.

Calories: 280
Fat: 3 grams
Carbohydrates: 46 grams
Protein: 16 grams
Sodium: 790 mg
Salt shakes: 20

DANGER ZONE: Sodium can hide in strange places in sandwich shops. At Subway, the 6-inch roasted garlic bread has 1,260 mg of sodium. That's more than half of the recommended daily maximum. That's just the bread on its own!

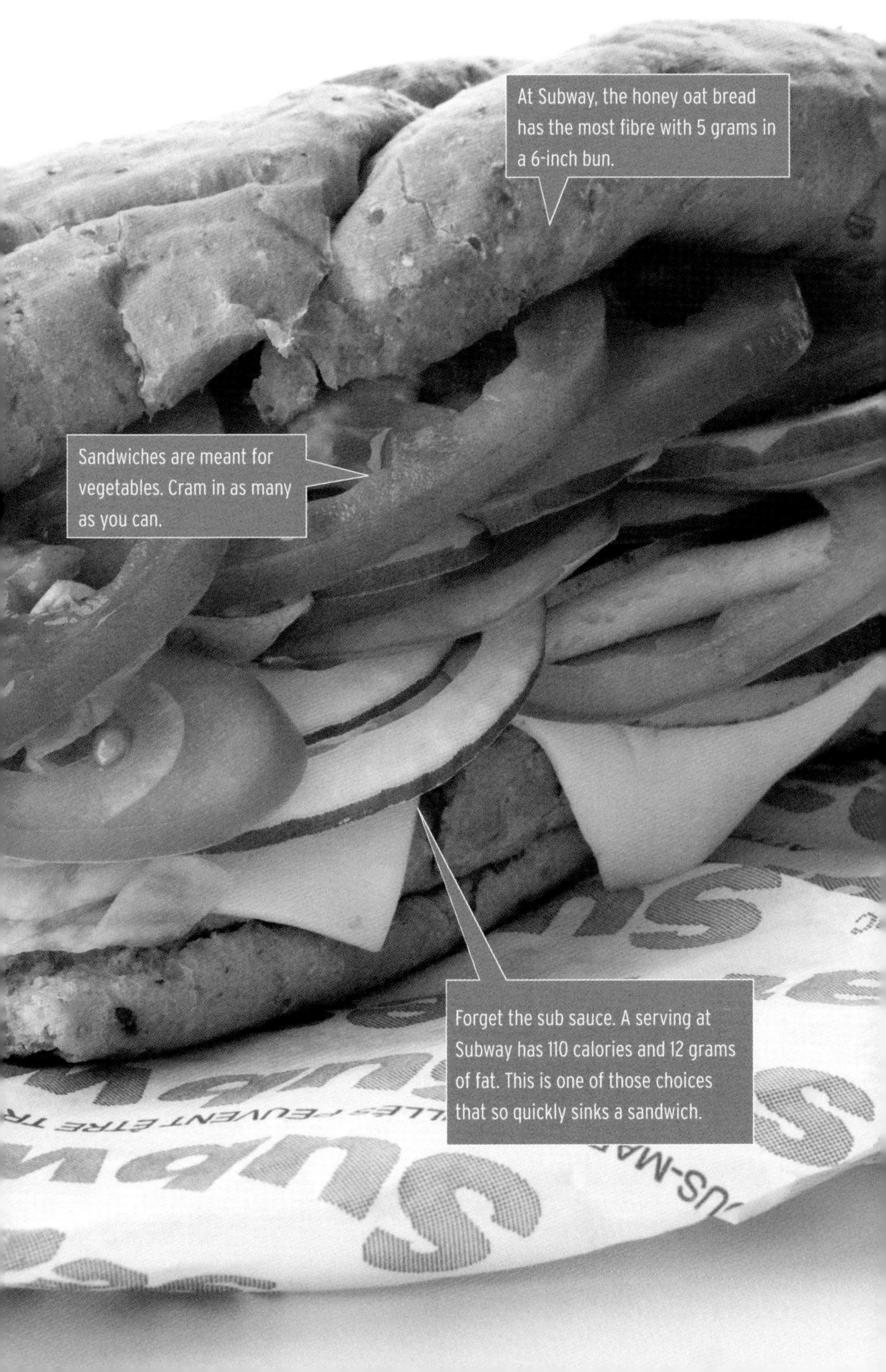
At Subway, the honey oat bread has the most fibre with 5 grams in a 6-inch bun.
Sandwiches are meant for vegetables. Cram in as many as you can.
Forget the sub sauce. A serving at Subway has 110 calories and 12 grams of fat. This is one of those choices that so quickly sinks a sandwich.

Best bets at the food court

The food court can be a minefield of fatty fare and sodium-soaked combos. But it is possible to make careful picks and walk away unharmed.

At Culture's

The dish: 3-Salad Combo, made with three-bean salad, beet salad, and orzo-and-sundried-tomato pasta salad.

The verdict: You will feel virtuous for piling a takeout tray with three kinds of salads. But this particular salad combo has 840 calories, 52 grams of fat and 2,410 mg of sodium. That's no different, nutritionally, than a colossal burger combo from most fast-food joints.

The swap: Pick your salads wisely. Choose just one of the hearty salads—the bean salad, for example, has 410 calories, 23 grams of fat and 970 mg of sodium—then ask your server to fill the remainder of the tray with the restaurant's lightest salads. The 45-calorie fruit salad is a great choice. So is the broccoli and cauliflower salad with its 60 calories and 3 grams of fat.

At Manchu Wok

The dish: Garden Plate

The verdict: It sounds like healthy fare, but the spread of mixed vegetables, noodles and fried rice has 910 calories, 40 grams of fat and a shocking 2,540 mg of sodium. That's half your day's worth of calories and fat and 10% more than the maximum amount of sodium health professionals say you should consume in a day.

The swap: Skip the combos and order off the à la carte menu. On its own, the Mixed Vegetables entree has 140 calories, 10 grams of fat and 510 mg of sodium. The Pineapple Chicken, made with marinated chicken, celery, green and red pepper and pineapple chunks has 160 calories, 8 grams of fat and just 250 mg of sodium.

At Taco Time

The dish: Beef and cheese burrito

The verdict: This beef-stuffed burrito has 556 calories, 25 grams of fat and 1,430 mg of sodium. While the calories are reasonable for a meal, it contains as much sodium as your body requires in a day.

The swap: Switch out the beef for beans to cut calories, slash sodium and keep the belly-filling protein. A Super Bean Burrito has 371 calories, 12 grams of fat and 584 mg of sodium.

At Vanellis

The dish: One slice of Roasted Vegetable Pesto Pizza

The verdict: With 600 calories and 33 grams of fat, this seemingly healthy slice of pizza has more calories than any other on the pizza menu. It also has 1,080 mg of sodium—two-thirds of your day's allotment.

The swap: Create your own pasta dish with whole-wheat pasta, marinara sauce and a selection of veggies for about 450 calories, 5 grams of fat and 600 mg of sodium.

THAI EXPRESS PAD THAI

With its bright green decor, emphasis on fresh ingredients and the cute take-out containers, it seems like Thai Express would serve only healthy dishes. But this version of the iconic Thai dish is mostly noodles fried with sauce, some chicken and a scant few vegetables.

THAI EXPRESS PAD THAI

Calories: 1,130

Fat: 40 grams

Carbohydrates: 160 grams

Protein: 33 grams

Sodium: 2,594 mg

Salt shakes: 65

MICHELINA'S CHEESE TORTELLINI (PER TRAY)

Calories: 330

Fat: 15 grams

Carbohydrates: 38 grams

Protein: 12 grams

Sodium: 880 mg

Salt shakes: 22

SMART SWAPS: It's hard to know what a smart swap would be, since Thai Express doesn't post nutrition information. But it's probably best to take a pass on foods made in the wok. Opt for soup and fresh foods, including the spring rolls served with peanut sauce and mango salad.

1 Thai Express Pad Thai

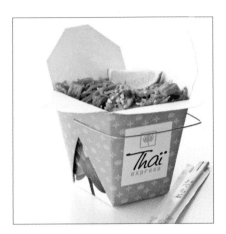

EQUALS

4 trays of Michelina's cheese tortellini

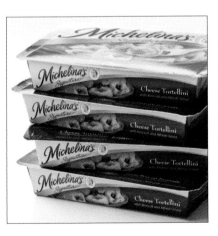

The Thai Express meal has the same number of calories as four trays of Michelina's cheese tortellini with broccoli and alfredo sauce.

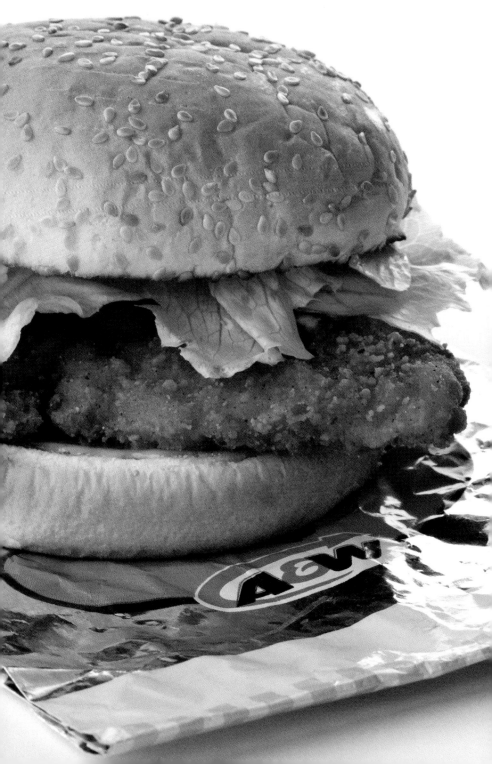

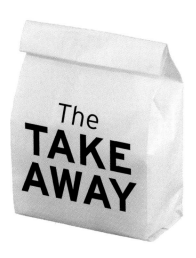

The TAKE AWAY

Get your fast food freshly made. That way you can make smart swaps and have some control over the toppings. You also know your food hasn't been sitting under a heat lamp for hours.

Don't get sucked into ordering a combo, whether you're at a burger joint, pizza parlour or food court. A meal deal might save you some pennies, but the discount won't make up for the few hundred extra—mostly empty—calories you'll end up downing without much notice.

Garnish wisely to cut back on calories, fat and sodium.

Pile on the veggies. Vegetables are scarce in the fast-food world. When you find them, get as many as you can.

Forget the fries. You don't have to omit them every time you pull through the drive-thru. But skipping a medium order of fries every week could help you lose about 6 pounds over the course of a year.

Go smaller instead of supersizing. Ordering the junior versions of burgers, fries and drinks can cut a fast-food meal's calorie count in half.

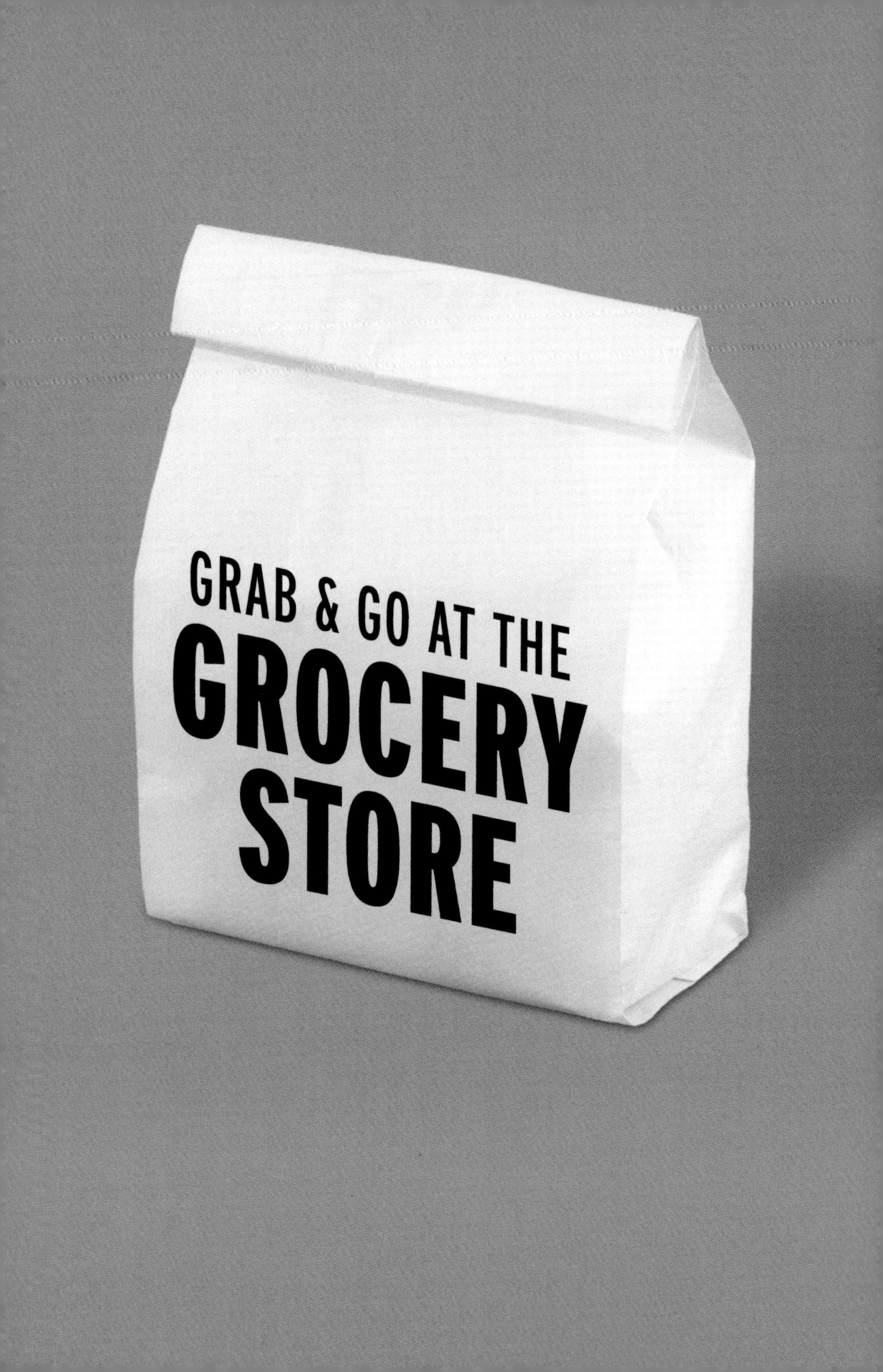

GRAB & GO AT THE
GROCERY
STORE

Grocery stores have gone from stocking ingredients to supplying complete meals. In this age of superstore supermarkets, you can get away with never having to cook.

A grocery store may seem a healthier place to get a meal than a greasy spoon. And many times it is. But depending where you push the shopping cart, that's not always the case.

Where to find the best grab-and-go meals at the grocery store

Walk over to

The salad section. It will have one of the most nutritious selections outside of your own kitchen. Pick a salad with dark greens, colourful vegetables and only a smattering of the yummy extras, like those crispy noodles and candied nuts.

The sandwich counter. Look for ones made with whole-wheat bread and lots of veggies. Be wary of premade sandwiches with creamy salad fillings. It's best if your grocery store, like the neighbourhood sub shop, custom makes your sandwich.

The produce section. Pick up a pair of hard-boiled eggs, a small green salad and a piece of fruit. Then take a trip past the bakery for a small whole-wheat roll. You can't get a more wholesome lunch.

Proceed with caution around

The deli. Those prepared potato and pasta salads are quick and tasty. But the calories will swiftly rack up with each bite.

Soups. Some are nutritious. Some are treacherous. Look for a broth-based soup with chunks of vegetables and beans or lentils. Creamy soups can be loaded with fat and little nutrition.

Premade pizza. Steer clear of pizzas that look like cardboard and are topped with tiny chips of obligatory vegetables and too many rounds of pepperoni. They won't taste good, and they're not good for you. Choose a thin-crust pizza that has lots of vegetables. Augment it with precut veggie spears or salad.

Rotisserie chicken. That roast chicken that looks like it came out of your oven has been spiked with sodium.

Walk right past

The hot deli section. Everything behind the glass—the wings, the chicken pieces, the potato wedges—is most likely deep-fried. You'll do so much better by going a few steps beyond this enticing fare. If you feel your willpower faltering, take a peek at the grease coating the bottom of the serving pans.

The bakery. With its pizza buns, chocolate croissants and mega-muffins—many with more than 400 calories each—it's nearly impossible to find a snack-sized treat in the bakery section. If you can't split a baked good, it's best to avoid temptation. Want something sweet? Buy a bar of dark chocolate—preferably one with more than 70% cocoa—and savour one or two squares after your meal. The rich taste will satisfy for about 100 calories.

Loblaws mixed fruit yogurt parfait

A yogurt parfait can be light and nutritious. But it can also be a deceiving food, one that appears healthy but is crammed with calories.

Loblaws doesn't provide nutrition numbers for many of its grab-and-go fare, but our tests reveal a sensible parfait. It easily slips under the 400 calorie target we should aim for in a breakfast, and its sodium is only 10% of your daily maximum. With 15 grams of protein, the parfait will keep you going until lunch. The chopped fruit is packed with fibre and antioxidants, and the yogurt provides a good dose of bone-building nutrients.

Calories: 385
Fat: 5 grams
Carbohydrates: 69 grams
Protein: 15 grams
Sodium: 231 mg
Salt shakes: 6

FARE WARNING: Some parfaits are swirled with sugar-sweetened fruit syrup, processed fruits and fatty granola, making them more like an ice cream sundae than a nutrient-rich meal. If there are no nutrition numbers to guide you, pick a parfait made with low-fat yogurt, real fruit chunks and just a smattering of granola.

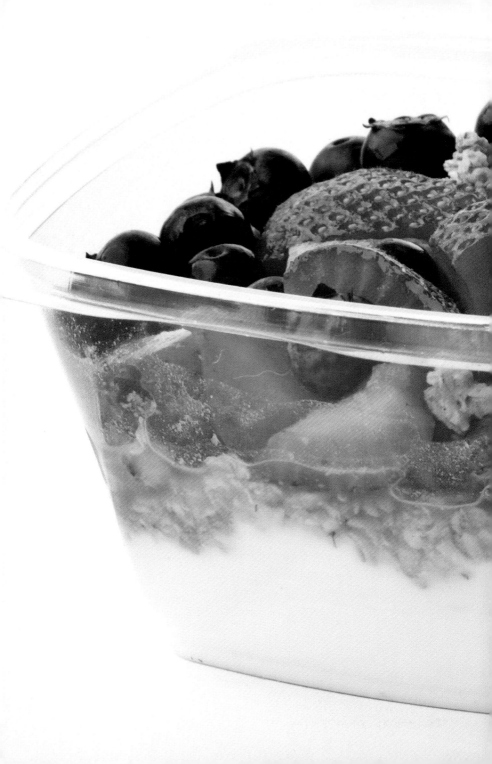

Sobeys slab birthday cake

In our mad-dash world, few of us have time to bake a cake from scratch, ice it and lovingly pipe on a message in picture-perfect cursive. Especially when the bakery at our local grocery store does it so well.

These days, the supermarket offers an impressive range of delectable desserts, from cupcakes to Black Forest cakes, from pecan pies to fruity flans. For birthdays, though, the classic chocolate slab cake continues to be one of the most popular pastries. It satisfies any age, from 8 to 88.

Serving size: 1 slice (1/6 cake)
Calories: 496
Fat: 23 grams
Carbohydrates: 66 grams
Protein: 6 grams
Sodium: 546 mg
Salt shakes: 14

SMART SWAP: Everyone loves sundaes, so it should be an easy swap. And you can still put a candle on top, light it and sing a rousing rendition of "Happy Birthday." A sundae made with 1/2 cup Compliments-brand French vanilla frozen yogurt, a 1/4 cup sliced strawberries, a drizzle of chocolate sauce and a fresh cherry on top has just 180 calories and 3 grams of fat. Plus you've saved yourself almost 500 mg of sodium.

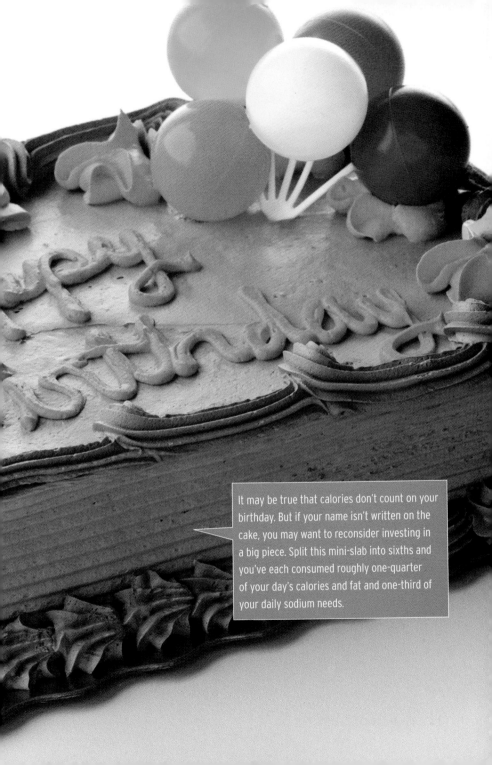

It may be true that calories don't count on your birthday. But if your name isn't written on the cake, you may want to reconsider investing in a big piece. Split this mini-slab into sixths and you've each consumed roughly one-quarter of your day's calories and fat and one-third of your daily sodium needs.

Bento Nouveau sushi

Sushi stands have popped up in many big grocery stores across Canada. That's good news for us Canucks, since a typical tray of sushi has fewer than 500 calories. And it's one of those dishes where you can see just about every ingredient: the wedge of avocado, the cluster of matchstick carrots and julienne cucumber, the slice of fish. Little is hidden in a piece of sushi. You know just what you're getting, and you can make a strong bet that it will be good for you.

Both of these sushi trays are considered lower-calorie, low-fat dishes by nutrition professionals—labels that are hard to achieve in the takeout world.

The fatty fish—it's recommended Canadians get two servings a week—provides a dose of heart-healthy omega-3 fats. And salmon is a good choice because it's a low-mercury fish.

Bento Nouveau often offers sushi made with brown rice. Consider this version the next time you buy sushi to get a little more whole grain in your daily diet. The switch from white rice will net you between 1 and 2 additional grams of fibre. It's not a big gain, but little swaps like this will add up over the course of a day.

FARE WARNING: Sushi laced with tempura or made with mayonnaise will have many more calories and much more fat. Keep your sushi simple and you'll pretty much be guaranteed that the nutrition numbers will be sane. Beware of dunking your sushi in too much salty soy sauce. One packet has about 500 mg of sodium—about one-third of the amount your body needs in a day.

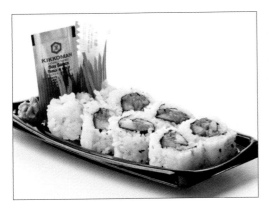

VEGETARIAN CALIFORNIA ROLL

Calories: 300

Fat: 5.5 grams

Carbohydrates: 58 grams

Protein: 7 grams

Sodium: 427 mg

Salt shakes: 11

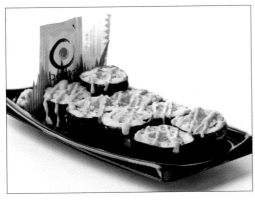

SPICY SALMON SUSHI ROLL

Calories: 350

Fat: 6 grams

Carbohydrates: 60 grams

Protein: 14 grams

Sodium: 691 mg

Salt shakes: 17

MEGAN'S TIP: If you are a sushi lover (like me), consider buying a bottle of low-sodium or light soy sauce to tuck in your desk drawer at the office. It's hard to find it in packets with takeout sushi trays. But it's a great swap, since the light version will typically have 25% less sodium than traditional soy sauce.

Loblaws salmon with mango sauce and wild rice pilaf

The portion size is perfect. The piece of salmon is about the size of the palm of your hand—just the way it should be—and delivers a dose of essential omega-3 fatty acids. The pilaf doesn't overwhelm the plate, like it does at so many restaurants. And the wild rice mixed in with the fluffy white grains brings a touch more fibre to the meal.

Round it out by getting a small green salad from the nearby produce section, making sure to pick the right pouch of dressing—say yes to a raspberry balsamic and no to a creamy Caesar.

Up the meal's nutrition and its elegance by scattering chopped fresh mango over the fish to get some vitamin C, beta carotene and additional fibre.

FARE WARNING: Not all hot plate items from Loblaws get such good reviews. Many have been deep-fried or sautéed in oil. Even the seemingly healthy rotisserie chicken can be a health hazard. A 150 gram serving has 525 mg of sodium—more than a third of what your body needs in a day.

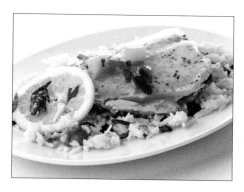

Calories: 332
Fat: 11 grams
Carbohydrates: 16 grams
Protein: 42 grams
Sodium: 580 mg
Salt shakes: 14 1/2

M&M Meat Shops butter chicken

At first glance—and compared with many restaurant meals—this tray of butter chicken, with its 410 calories and 17 grams of fat, seems very reasonable. But with 800 mg of sodium and 10 grams of saturated fat—both half your daily allotment—the meal begins to slide. Plus it has only 2 grams of fibre; you'd have to scramble the rest of the day to meet the recommended quota. Another of this dish's downfalls is its lack of discernible vegetables. Adding on a serving of M&M's Bean and Carrot Medley will help.

SMART SWAP: For an equally decadent chicken dish, pick up M&M's Bistro Chicken Portobello and pair it with its Rice and Vegetable Medley and a double serving of its grilled vegetables. The stuffed chicken breast with the sides has just 320 calories, 4.5 grams of fat and 720 mg of sodium.

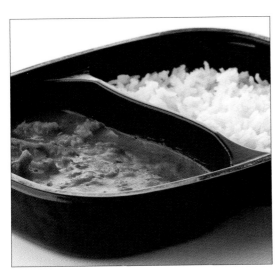

Per 340 gram serving
Calories: 410
Fat: 17 grams
Carbohydrates:
    44 grams
Protein: 19 grams
Sodium: 800 mg
Salt shakes: 20

Sobeys garlic bread

Few people will turn down a piece of toasty cheesy garlic bread. The premade appetizer, found at just about every grocery store, is a popular pickup for a potluck party or a family spaghetti dinner. Unfortunately, the ease of getting the garlic loaf to the table is the only thing going for it.

Serving size: entire loaf
Calories: 1,108
Fat: 57 grams
Carbohydrates: 110 grams
Protein: 38 grams
Sodium: 2,419 mg
Salt shakes: 60

SMART SWAP: Walk past the garlic bread and grab a fresh store-made loaf of whole-grain bread. At home, pop it into the oven for a few minutes to warm it up. Then dip one or two slices into extra-virgin olive oil mixed with balsamic vinegar. If you can't give up the garlic, add a piece of a fresh-pressed clove into the oil to get that garlicky zing.

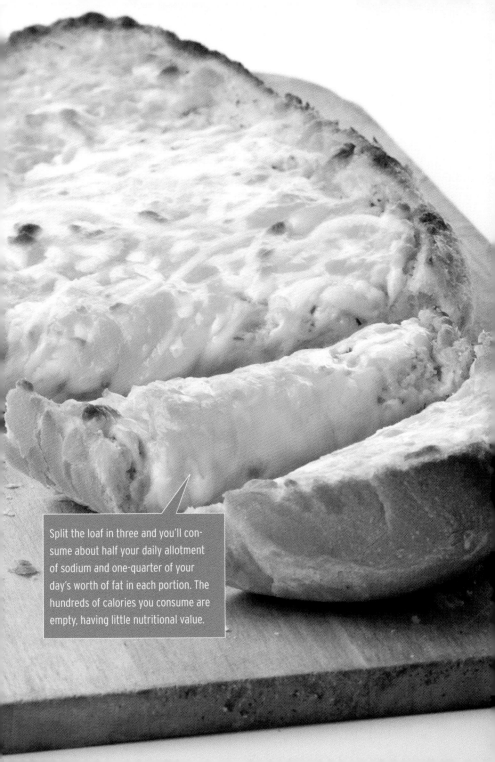

Split the loaf in three and you'll consume about half your daily allotment of sodium and one-quarter of your day's worth of fat in each portion. The hundreds of calories you consume are empty, having little nutritional value.

Costco's chicken penne alfredo

A shopping trip to Costco can be both exhilarating and exhausting. After tramping kilometres through the sprawling warehouse and digging for deals, you may not want to go home and cook dinner for the family.

While the chicken penne alfredo is clearly not health food, its homemade look and chunks of white-meat chicken make it seem as though it's a better choice than a fast-food burger.

Serving size: 1/4 of tray
Calories: 568
Fat: 24 grams
Carbohydrates: 56 grams
Protein: 33 grams
Sodium: 1,156 mg
Salt shakes: 29

SMART SWAP: Go to the freezer section and pick up Costco's brand (that's Kirkland Signature) of thin-crust cheese pizza. A quarter of the pie has 330 calories and 14 grams of fat. Serve it toasty from the oven with a portion of Costco's apple cranberry pecan salad, which is packed with nutrient-rich whole foods.

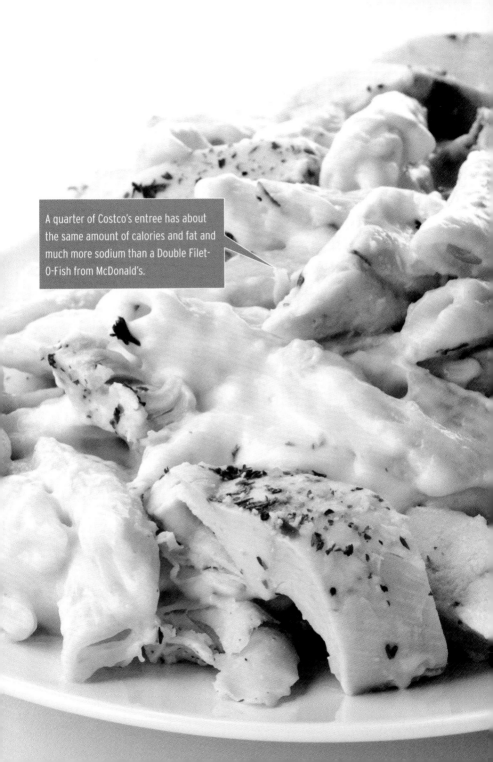

A quarter of Costco's entree has about the same amount of calories and fat and much more sodium than a Double Filet-O-Fish from McDonald's.

How to shop like a pro

Shannon Crocker, a registered dietitian with 17 years of experience, is a foodie who likes grocery shopping, trying new foods and creating recipes. At home, she battles a husband and two young sons about what constitutes a serving of vegetables. Her favourite food is fresh, summer-harvested tomatoes—in just about everything.

Everyone has good intentions of making meals at home. We all know preparing dishes yourself is the best way to control calories and boost nutrition. But some days, time is at a premium. When do you find yourself dashing to the grocery store for a quick meal?
Like most people juggling work and a busy family schedule, the dash happens in the five minutes after work ends when I realize I've got nothing meal-worthy in the fridge and I have to get the kids to their activities for 6 p.m.

Do you have a go-to meal to take home to the family?
In a hurry, our go-to meal is a big veggie tray and the wood-oven, thin-crust pizza served at the grab-and-go section of our local grocery store. Mine is loaded with veggies and the men in the house get plain cheese.

I also love quick at-home assembly meals. At the store, I'll grab a variety of healthy ingredients that we can throw together for make-your-own wraps or do-it-yourself salads. That way everyone in the family gets something they like, and I don't have to make it all.

If I'm looking for a quick bite for myself, I go for the salads. Sometimes I get sandwiches made—but only if I can get them made to order with good, fresh ingredients and whole-grain breads.

Sushi is also a good bet—I like the brown rice sushi—just go light on the soy sauce.

What about snacks for after your son's soccer game?

Whoa! Sore point here. I've seen a lot of kids with sugary, punch-like drinks and gummies as a post-game treat. I may not be popular with orange wedges, mini-muffins and water, but this is sports, and I think that should go hand in hand with healthy foods.

Where is the grocery store's minefield—the place where you should tread carefully?

Step lightly in the ready-to-go hot meal section. Those food choices might smell great when you walk in at the end of the day, and they're quick, but so many are loaded with salt and fat. That includes the all-in-one meals packaged in one simple box. Rarely is something that is really good for you going to come with a pull-tab and directions to heat at 375 degrees for 30 minutes.

Where is the place where you can't really go wrong?

No one will be surprised by my answer: the fresh produce section. There are so many prepared vegetables that can help make meal time a breeze. Like the precut veggie mixes that you can use to whip up a stir-fry, or the salads that you can build a meal around. I love the cut-up squash, to make a quick soup.

How about for a treat? Dietitians do sometimes indulge, right?

Who doesn't like a little chocolate? Really, was there another answer? I go for a square of dark chocolate, a few chocolate almonds or melted chocolate drizzled over berries.

Walmart's Buffalo chicken skewers and potato salad

At Walmart's grocery superstores, shoppers can pick up their evening meal along with their office supplies, pet food, toilet paper and packages of tube socks.

From roast chicken to trays of lasagna, Walmart will likely have that ready-to-go meal you need. If barbeque fare is on your list, you might pick up a pack of grill-ready chicken skewers and a tub of potato salad.

I've learned that it's pretty easy to build a leafy salad at Walmart (and other grocery stores), so now I bypass the prepared salad section, which mostly stocks creamy, noodle-y salads. I buy a box of mixed prewashed greens—the darker the better—a pack of prewashed and sliced mushrooms and a container of cherry tomatoes. Minutes after you get home home, all the ingredients can be tossed together in a big bowl with fancy, bottled balsamic vinaigrette. With a half sandwich or small, hearty wrap, it's the perfect grab-and-go meal.

SMART SWAPS: Skewers and premade salads don't have to be off the Walmart menu. Scrap the seasoned chicken and buy the plain chicken and vegetable skewers. You'll save about 450 mg of sodium per skewer. And choose a real salad—you know, one with actual vegetables—for your side.

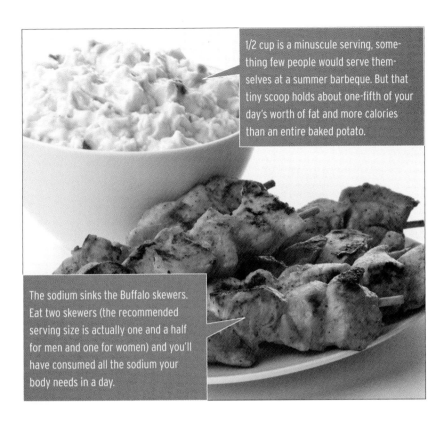

1/2 cup is a minuscule serving, something few people would serve themselves at a summer barbeque. But that tiny scoop holds about one-fifth of your day's worth of fat and more calories than an entire baked potato.

The sodium sinks the Buffalo skewers. Eat two skewers (the recommended serving size is actually one and a half for men and one for women) and you'll have consumed all the sodium your body needs in a day.

PKG. OF 5 SKEWERS

Calories: 557

Fat: 11 grams

Carbohydrates: 0 grams

Protein: 114 grams

Sodium: 3,031 mg

Salt shakes: 76

1 SKEWER

Calories: 111

Fat: 2 grams

Carbohydrates: 0 grams

Protein: 23 grams

Sodium: 606 mg

Salt shakes: 15

1/2 CUP RESER'S BRAND POTATO SALAD

Calories: 220

Fat: 13 grams

Carbohydrates: 24 grams

Protein: 2 grams

Sodium: 530 mg

Salt shakes: 13

Freezer finds

Having a well-stocked freezer means you don't always have to dash to the grocery store when your fridge is bare. With the right frozen foods, a dinner of baked salmon, warm whole-wheat bread and roasted mixed vegetables can be on your table in just 25 minutes. That's not much longer than it would take to drive to the store, find parking, stand in line to order the food and pay and then rush home. And while the food is cooking in the oven, you'll have time to slice lemon for the salmon, put out a dish of olive oil for the bread, set the table—and maybe even light a candle.

You can whip up a quick and tasty meal with President's Choice Blue Menu Atlantic salmon skinless fillets, Ace Bakery Bake Your Own Multigrain Petits Pains and Europe's Best Roasted Gourmet Tuscan Inspired Blend of roasted potatoes, onions, zucchini, red peppers and eggplant. One salmon fillet contains 250 calories, 15 grams of fat, 85 mg of sodium and 28 grams of protein. Three slices of bread have 130 calories, 1.5 grams of fat, 26 grams of carbohydrates (including 3 grams of fibre), 4 grams of protein and 230 mg of sodium. And a cup of roasted veggies offers up 100 calories, 2 grams of fat, 20 grams of carbohydrates (including 2 grams of fibre), 2 grams of protein and just 10 mg of sodium.

Total meal for one
Calories: 480
Fat: 18.5 grams
Carbohydrates: 46 grams (including 5 grams fibre)
Protein: 34 grams
Sodium: 325 mg
Salt shakes: 8

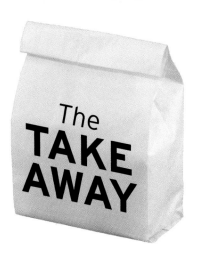

The
TAKE AWAY

Choose meals made with foods as close to their natural state as possible. A grocery store has a plethora of good options—you just have to find them.

Limit meals made with prepackaged, highly processed foods with long lists of ingredients you can't pronounce. Grocery stores are packed with these, too.

Be creative with grab-and-go meals. Look past the prepared foods and collect whole-food items, such as hard-boiled eggs, fruit, small whole-wheat rolls and yogurt, to build your own lunch or dinner.

Consider adding a premade or boxed salad to every meal you pick up. If your entree lacks something nutritionally, leafy greens will help make up those deficiencies.

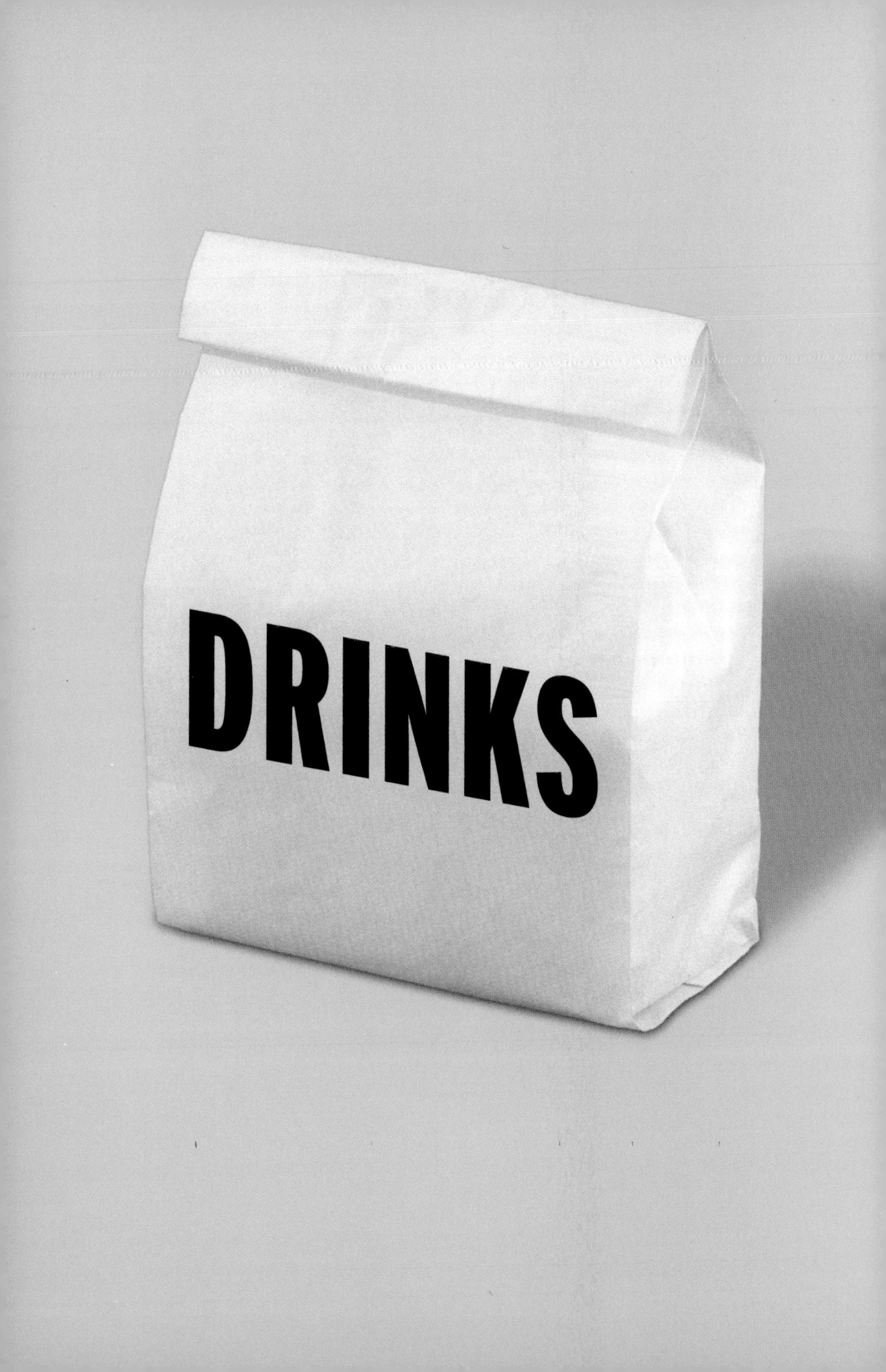
DRINKS

A frosty iced coffee on a hot summer's day. A slushy smoothie after a long bout of yoga. A sweet, fruity iced tea during an afternoon break from work. Few things taste as delicious as a drink that's quenching your thirst. It can be hard to remember, mid-satisfying gulp, that you are drinking down calories, sometimes at an alarming rate.

When it comes to beverages, you rarely have to worry about fat and salt (unless you regularly drink those elaborate coffeehouse concoctions—then watch out). Rather, the main nutrition concern with drinks is the calories that come from sugar. There is an astonishing abundance of the sweet stuff in many of our drinks. Start looking. You'll be frightened.

Juice

In judicious amounts, 100% juice can definitely be part of a healthy diet. Along with that rise-and-shine taste, a glass of juice contains important vitamins, minerals and antioxidants. But if you regularly slurp juice instead of water, those benefits are quickly wiped out by all the calories contained in the glass.

Size matters

Like with so many foods, it's the amount of what you consume that's important. According to Canada's Food Guide, a serving of juice is a 1/2 cup. The next time you reach into the fridge for OJ, pour out a 1/2 cup in a measuring glass, just to see how small that serving is. It will seem minute because we've become accustomed to the bulky bottles sold as single servings. Consider that a 355 mL bottle of real orange juice has about 150 calories—the equivalent of three store-bought chocolate-chip cookies. The weight will creep on if you drink a bottle every day.

The Good Old Days: Can't give up your juice habit? Find a set of old-time juice glasses from the 1960s to use for your morning OJ. These diminutive cups will likely hold the recommended 1/2 cup serving size and contain enough to get your taste buds going in the morning. This way, you can satisfy your juice cravings for about 50 calories a day.

Fake juice

Fruit cocktail. Fruit drink. Fruit beverage. These labels mean that you're drinking fruit-flavoured sugar water, not juice. It also means that the nutritional benefits found in the fresh-squeezed stuff are now gone. Scour the fine print and you'll see the first three ingredients will likely be water, fruit juice from concentrate and sugar. Not necessarily in that order.

Juice at a glance

Brand (355 mL serving)	Calories	Sugar (grams)	Sugar (teaspoons)
Arizona fruit punch	147	37	9
Fruitopia Strawberry Passion Awareness	175	42	10
Minute Maid Five Alive Citrus	170	40	9 1/2
Tim Hortons orange juice	166	39	9
V8 Splash Berry Blend	165	40	9 1/2

Ocean Spray cranberry cocktail

Cranberry cocktail will almost always be loaded with added sugars. Try a raw cranberry and you'll see why—and how much—sugar needs to be added to make this ruby-hued drink taste so good.

Serving size: 355 mL
Calories: 185
Carbohydrates: 44 grams (all sugars)
Sodium: 48 mg
Salt shakes: 1

MEGAN'S TIP: I no longer drink my juice straight up. So I've started diluting 100% juice with sparkling water, about one part juice to three parts water. It's a great gourmet drink. I like it better than pop and know I'm getting some nutritional benefit for few calories. Try it with orange or grapefruit juice, peach nectar or pineapple juice. Or try it with cherry juice—my favourite.

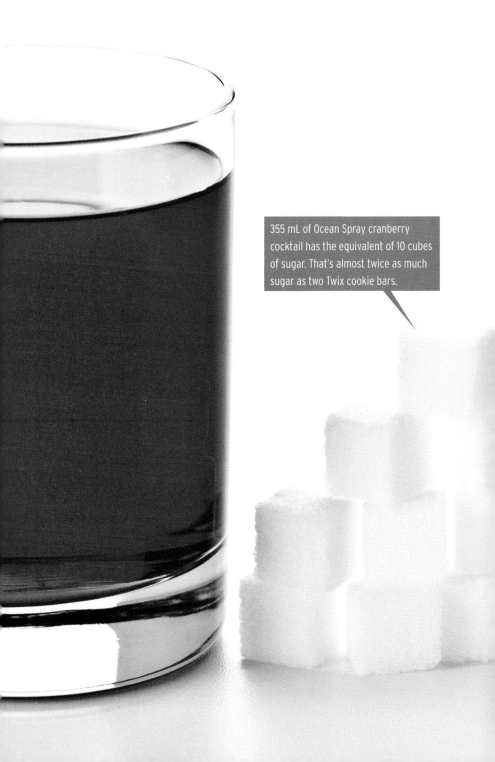

355 mL of Ocean Spray cranberry cocktail has the equivalent of 10 cubes of sugar. That's almost twice as much sugar as two Twix cookie bars.

Pop

Imagine dumping 9 teaspoons of sugar over the top of your morning bowl of cereal. Repellent, right? That's how much sugar lurks inside a typical can of pop.

Like any food, pop can be a once-in-a-while treat without causing much concern. The problem is that most Canadians drink 82 litres of pop a year. Some might consider the never-ending sugar high a national crisis.

Size matters

When our parents sipped pop as a treat, they likely put their straw in an 8-ounce (250 mL) glass bottle. These days, single-serving cans—pretty much the smallest option available—contain 12 ounces, or 355 mL, of soda. More commonly, people reach for a bottle of pop because it's priced at a better value. These supersize containers often hold as much as 700 mL of pop. That's 300 calories of the sugary stuff.

Sugar-free

Diet pops provide that sort-of-soda taste without the calorie consequence. Health Canada has approved five sugar substitutes for use in food and beverages, and research has shown that they likely aren't health hazards. But you have to decide if you're willing to swap calories for artificial sweeteners.

Pop at a glance

Brand (355 mL serving)	Calories	Sugar (grams)	Sugar (teaspoons)
A&W root beer	195	51	12
Canada Dry ginger ale	142	34	8
Coca-Cola	140	39	9
C'plus orange	130	35	8
7UP	160	42	10

A Soda Too Far: If you love soda, consider limiting yourself to one can of pop a week. Even this is hard to defend, since the drink provides no nutritional benefit. But consider that drinking a 150 calorie can of soda every day for a year equals a 15-pound increase in weight. Which means . . . give up your daily soda habit and you could lose 15 pounds this year.

7-Eleven Cream Soda Slurpee

Okay, this is the most over-the-top example for soda pop. But the Slurpee *is* incredibly popular. People line up for the slushy treat on hot summer days. And the drink is so famous it has its own crafty straw designed to help its fans scoop up every last bit of Slurpee at the bottom of the cup. Even though ice is one of its main components, the Slurpee is incredibly, exceedingly sweet.

Serving size: 800mL
Calories: 383
Carbohydrates: 99 grams (including 97 grams sugars)
Sodium: 146 mg
Salt shakes: 4

SMART SWAP: If you are dying for a drink of super sweet cream soda, grabbing a can of the pink-hued pop from the cooler is a better bet. Sipping a Crush cream soda straight up, rather than in Slurpee form, will save you about half the calories and half the sugar. Or consider a Creamsicle instead of a cream soda to satisfy your sweet tooth on a hot summer day. The classic frozen treat has 70 calories, less than a gram of fat and 13 grams of sugar—that's 84 grams less than what's in a frosty pink Slurpee.

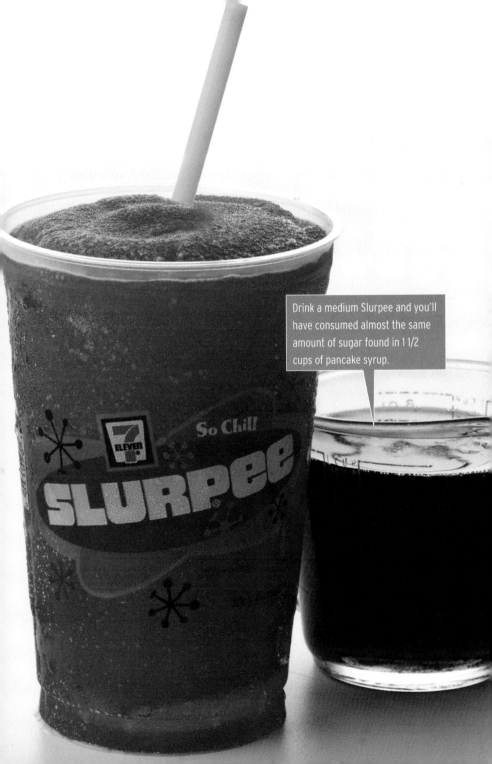

Drink a medium Slurpee and you'll have consumed almost the same amount of sugar found in 1 1/2 cups of pancake syrup.

Iced tea

Tea is the second most popular drink in the world. Water ranks first.

In its unadulterated form, tea has everything going for it: a soothing, familiar taste; it's natural—there's nothing artificial about it; it has a host of health benefits; and it is calorie-free.

When tea is on ice, you get all of those things—plus a refreshing, cool drink on a hot day. Too bad, then, that when you buy iced tea in a bottle or get a glass at a restaurant, you'll likely end up with a drink that has more sugar than tea in it.

Plain ole tea

Researchers around the world are investigating the health properties of tea. They are studying whether the antioxidants in tea protect against heart disease, impact cancer risk and reduce the risk of developing kidney stones.

The evidence is still being weighed. In the meantime, drinking unadorned tea can't hurt you. And it very likely does help.

Tea hybrids

Don't believe the hype. Pop mixed with tea is just gussied-up sugary, fizzy water. All the calories obliterate the health benefits of the tea.

A 355 mL can of Canada Dry white tea ginger ale with raspberry (phew) has 128 calories and 32.5 grams of sugar, the equivalent of eight sugar cubes rattling around in the can.

Iced tea at a glance

Brand (355 mL serving)	Calories	Sugar (grams)	Sugar (teaspoons)
Arizona green tea with ginseng and honey	99	25	6
Lipton PureLeaf iced tea, lemon flavour	105	26	6
Nestea iced tea	114	28	6 1/2
Snapple peach green tea	120	31	7
Tim Hortons lemon iced tea	110	27	6 1/2

Arizona iced tea with raspberry flavour

This colossal can of iced tea is one of the sweetest you'll find at the convenience store. Sugar-wise, slurping it down is like eating six popsicles in one sitting.

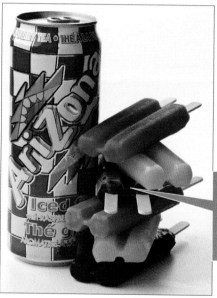

Serving size: 695 mL

Calories: 250

Carbohydrates: 69 grams
   (including 67 grams sugars)

Sodium: 28 mg

Salt shakes: <1

This humongous 695 mL serving of iced tea has 250 calories and 67 grams of sugar—the equivalent of 16 teaspoons.

SMART SWAP: There's no need for tea to be loaded with this much sugar. If you're on the road and looking for a gentle iced pick-me-up, head to a coffee house where a barista can make you a lovely iced concoction by pouring freshly brewed tea over ice. If you like it a little sweet, add in one pack of sugar for just 15 calories. You'll get all of tea's benefits without the nasty sugar spike.

HOLD THE CREAM

1 Harvey's chocolate milkshake

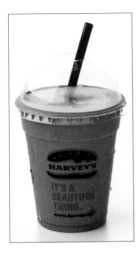

Calories: 730

Fat: 33 grams

Carbohydrates: 91 grams (including 78 grams
sugars)

Protein: 17 grams

Sodium: 520 mg

Salt shakes: 13

EQUALS

2 1/2 cups of whipped topping

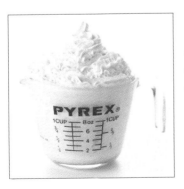

**A 730 calorie milkshake sounds
over-the-top. But would you guess
that it has as much fat as 2 1/2
cups of whipped topping?**

Rockstar energy drink

Energy drinks are the latest blockbuster beverage to hit store shelves. There seem to be a zillion and one varieties, all sold in bold, brightly coloured cans with many exclamation-marked claims touting their ability to give you extra powers.

Yes, they have caffeine and other mood enhancers. But you will also feel a surge after downing an energy drink because of the many teaspoons of sugar swirling inside the can.

ROCKSTAR ENERGY DRINK
Serving size: 473 mL can
Calories: 280
Carbohydrates: 62 grams (all sugars)
Sodium: 80 mg
Salt shakes: 2

FAST FACT: Clearly energy drinks are here to stay. More and more varieties—ones spiked with juice or laced with coffee—fill coolers at convenience stores. Although Health Canada has approved them, it has put a cap on the amount of caffeine the drinks can contain—180 mg in a single serving, about the equivalent amount of caffeine found in a medium coffee. Researchers at Harvard, arguably the smartest folks on earth, recommend ditching them from your diet.

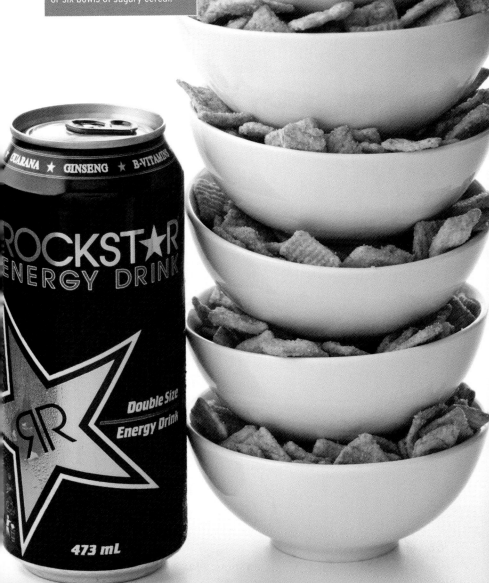

Among the most sugary out there, Rockstar's original energy drink has 62 grams of sugar—the equivalent of 15 sugar cubes or six bowls of sugary cereal.

STARBUCKS GRANDE ICED PEPPERMINT WHITE CHOCOLATE MOCHA

Fancy coffee drinks can range from low-cal treats to diet-destroying indulgences. It all depends on what you choose to put in—and on—your swanky cup of joe.

At Starbucks, a grande iced non-fat café latte has just 90 calories. But use 2% milk, add in peppermint and white chocolate mocha flavourings and top it with whipped cream and the same size iced coffee has 500 calories, 20 grams of fat and 69 grams of sugar. That's an over-the-top coffee concoction.

Made with 2% milk and topped with whipped cream
Calories: 500
Fat: 20 grams
Carbohydrates: 73 grams (including 69 grams sugars)
Protein: 10 grams
Sodium: 180 mg
Salt shakes: 4 1/2

HOLD THE CREAM: Most coffee shops let you custom make your drink. Order your fancy coffee with non-fat or low-fat milk and get it half-sweet (the barista will use just half the usual amount of flavouring) to cut as many as 200 calories. Skipping the whipped topping can also save as many as 100 calories and 10 grams of fat.

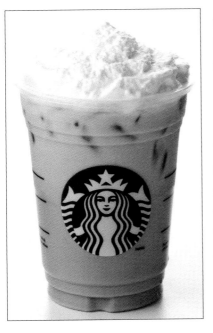

1 Starbucks Grande
Iced Peppermint White
Chocolate Mocha

This drink made with 2% milk and topped with whipped cream has the same amount of sugar as four and a half marshmallow dream bars from Starbucks.

EQUALS

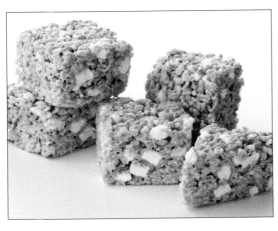

4 1/2 Starbucks
Marshmallow
Dream Bars

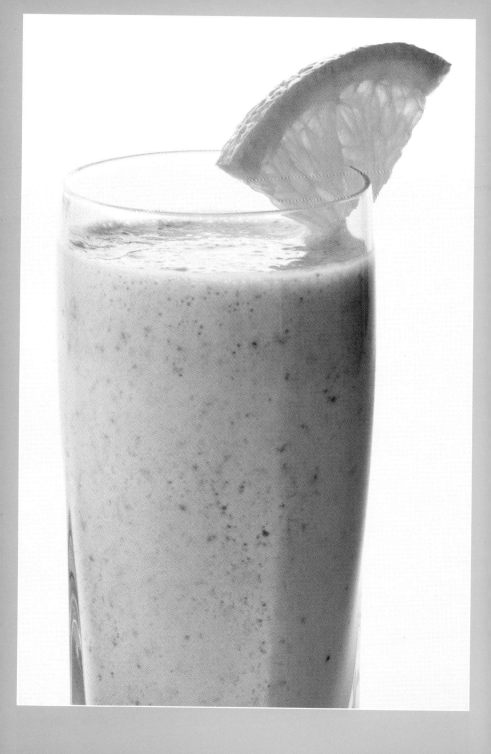

Smoothies

Smoothies have been touted as a well-rounded breakfast in a glass. Sometimes, this nutrition claim is true. Other times, smoothies are loaded with calories and sugar. They're another one of those foods that need to be carefully scrutinized before you start merrily slurping up the icy drink.

At Booster Juice

The Strawberry Sunshine smoothie, made with strawberries, passion fruit, guava, bananas and yogurt, has 315 calories, less than 1 gram of fat and 3 grams of protein.

The Canadian Colada, made with pineapples, coconut, bananas and vanilla frozen yogurt, has 455 calories, 7 grams of fat and 8 grams of protein.

The Funky Monkey, made with banana, chocolate soy milk and vanilla frozen yogurt, contains 585 calories, almost 9 grams of fat and 20 grams of protein.

At Jugo Juice

The Raspberry Rush smoothie, made with raspberries, strawberries, cranberry juice and low-fat yogurt, has 286 calories, 2.7 grams of fat and 4.4 grams of protein.

The Pomegranate Protein smoothie , made with whey protein, blackberries, banana, low-fat frozen yogurt and pomegranate juice, has 411 calories, 4.6 grams of fat and 26.6 grams of protein.

The Banana Buzz smoothie, made with banana, mocha iced coffee and low-fat frozen yogurt, has 510 calories, 10.9 grams of fat and 4.7 grams of protein.

Homemade strawberry banana smoothie

Smoothies are a breeze to make at home. A quick whirl with the blender will en-sure you have a healthy, relatively low-calorie drink. And it will likely cost many dollars less than store-bought. (The toasted wheat germ adds a little extra fibre.)

1/2 cup frozen, sliced strawberries

1 medium frozen banana, cut into chunks

1 cup 1% milk

1/2 cup 1% Greek-style plain yogurt

1 tablespoon toasted wheat germ

In a blender, buzz together all ingredients. Pour into a tall glass and enjoy.

This simple, nutritious recipe makes one large smoothie.

Calories: 346
Fat: 4.5 grams
Protein: 19 grams

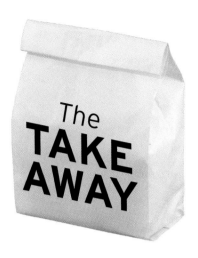

The
TAKE AWAY

Scrutinize labels. There will usually be more calories
and sugar than you'd figure.

Size matters. Just as a massive burger contains
many more calories than the junior version, a gargantuan can of
iced tea will likely hold a gigantic number of calories.

Use small, special glasses for your favourite juices
(and other much-loved, calorie-rich drinks). Relish every sip.

Watch out for energy drinks. Yes, they contain caffeine.
But they are also crammed with sugar.

APPETIZERS

Appetizers. Starters. Hors d'oeuvres. The delightful tidbits that get your taste buds warmed up and ready for the entree.

Problem is, in most cases the preprandials are as big—calorie-wise—as the real meal. Make a poor pick and you'll lose the chance of eating healthy before your entree hits the table. Even the ones that sound sane can contain as many calories as a drive-thru burger.

There are sensible starters hiding in restaurant menus. But you have to look carefully to find them. Good luck. It's tricky work.

What to look for in an appetizer

Bite for bite, appetizers often pack more calories than any other item on the menu. It would be easy to preach skipping this part of the menu entirely.

But if it's a special occasion, or if the starters are your favourite part of dining out, you don't have to sidestep them. It is possible to find a pre-entree indulgence that won't capsize your whole meal.

Look for
- Items that are fruit or vegetable based. Fresh spring rolls are almost always a sound choice.
- Grilled or broiled fish and shellfish. They serve up a lot of flavour for few calories.
- Clear soups, not the creamy kind. A cup of soup does dual duty by revving up your taste buds while curbing your appetite.
- Chicken, pork or beef satay to split with your dining companion.

Steer clear of
- Appetizers that come coated in calorie-laden sauces.
- Foods that have been dunked in a deep fryer. That seems obvious, but cooks can hide the fatty truth by using adjectives such as "crispy" or "lightly battered." Check with the server about how an appetizer is prepared.
- Anything with cheese as the main ingredient. It's very likely it will contain many calories per bite.
- If you are tracking your sodium intake, beware of pickled items and dishes made with soy sauce. These will be swimming in salt.

Ask about

- The size of a starter. Even the healthy ones can be as large as a meal. It's good to know ahead of time if you and your dining partner can happily share the calories.
- Dips and dressings. Can you get them on the side? That way you can control how much sauce—and how many calories—gets draped on your appetizer.
- Extra veggies. See if you can start your meal with chopped fruit or vegetable spears. These items may not be on the menu, but most restaurants are happy to accommodate requests.
- Substitutions. Ask if you can swap the accompanying flatbread for vegetable sticks if you've ordered the warm cheese spread or featured savoury dip.
- Cooking methods. Ask if you can get an appetizer baked or grilled instead of fried.

The Keg shrimp cocktail

It can be hard to locate a slimming choice in the meat-and-potato fare at the Keg. Especially when you're searching through the appetizers, where many selections clock in with more calories than a meal. But there is one standout starter: the shrimp cocktail. This classic steakhouse appetizer is elegantly short on calories. One of the reasons, surely, for its timeless appeal.

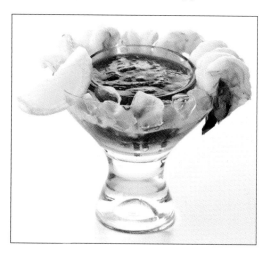

Calories: 127
Fat: 1 gram
Carbohydrates: 7 grams
Protein: 24 grams
Sodium: 823 mg
Salt shakes: 20 1/2

DANGER ZONE: The Keg's bruschetta contains 1,145 calories and 58 grams of fat, including 22 grams of saturated fat—more than what's in eight pats of butter. The French onion soup is a sodium tsunami with a staggering 2,667 mg of sodium—almost twice the amount your body needs in a day.

Red Lobster Cheddar Bay biscuits

At Red Lobster, the abundance of grilled seafood and fresh vegetable sides makes it easy to dine light.

While you're congratulating yourself for steering clear of the fried fare, make sure you also watch out for the Cheddar Bay biscuits. These complimentary buns, which pack lots of empty calories and next to no nutritional benefit, will quickly sink the ship.

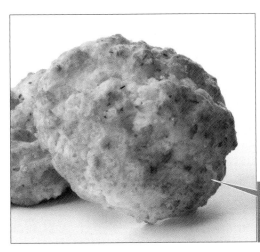

Serving size: 1 biscuit
Calories: 150
Fat: 8 grams
Carbohydrates: 16 grams
Protein: 3 grams
Sodium: 350 mg
Salt shakes: 9

Two biscuits have as many calories as two Twinkies and four more grams of fat.

DANGER ZONE: A pair of these biscuits contains one-quarter of your day's worth of fat and almost half of your daily sodium needs.

EAST SIDE MARIO'S CHEDDAR CHEESE STICKS

At East Side's, the starters have a real Italian-American flair. Chicken wings are dipped in garlic Parmesan sauce. Calamari comes *al diavolo*. And Budda Boomers—that's deep-fried pieces of pizza dough—arrive toasty hot and liberally sprinkled with Parmesan Romano.

It's easy to suspect these three items of being fatty fare. But other diet busters on East Side's starter menu are harder to spot. For example, the stuffed mushroom caps have a third of a day's worth of fat, while the bruschetta for two has almost as many calories as four slices of Mario's cheese pizza. Now, does that sound like a starter to you?

EAST SIDE MARIO'S CHEDDAR CHEESE STICKS
Calories: 470
Fat: 30.5 grams
Carbohydrates: 44 grams
Protein: 17 grams
Sodium: 2,050 mg
Salt shakes: 51 1/2

SMART SWAPS: Italian wedding soup. A bowl of this savoury broth, filled with mini-meatballs, spinach and confetti pasta, has just 90 calories and 4 grams of fat. The many spoonfuls of soup will likely satisfy as much as a few bites of gooey cheese—but for far fewer calories. Or consider ordering the bruschetta for one—but split it between two. You will get the enjoyment of a flavourful starter—and a dose of nutrient-rich tomatoes—for just 175 calories and about 9 grams of fat.

1 order of East Side Mario's cheddar cheese sticks

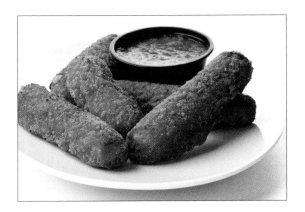

EQUALS

9 cups of cheese popcorn

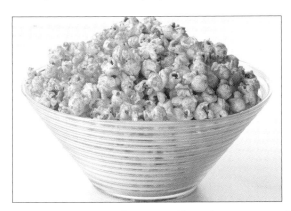

Mario's cheese stick appetizer has more calories and three times more sodium than 9 cups of cheese popcorn, and the same amount of fat.

EARLS KITCHEN & BAR
WARM SPINACH AND FETA DIP

Earls serves up sophisticated starters with an international flair. Your choices include sushi, tacos on white corn tortillas and chili chicken with crispy wontons.

With these appetizers, served on sleek white plates and beautifully decorated with swirls of sauce and edible greenery, it can be hard to spot the excess calories. Would you guess that the prawn dynamite roll has 445 calories and 20 grams fat—more calories and fat than what's found in a large order of fries from Harvey's?

The spinach and feta dip, made with aged cheddar, cream and feta cheeses, tries to camouflage its calories with spinach, artichokes and a healthy-sounding accompaniment of toasted flatbread. But despite the dip's green hue, this is a starter that needs to be split—many ways.

EARLS KITCHEN & BAR
WARM SPINACH AND FETA DIP
Calories: 942
Fat: 49 grams
Carbohydrates: 89 grams
Protein: 38 grams
Sodium: 2,066 mg
Salt shakes: 52

1 HOT DOG AND BUN
Calories: 200
Fat: 7 grams
Carbohydrates: 24 grams
Protein: 9 grams
Sodium: 650 mg
Salt shakes: 16

SMART SWAP: Get a salad. Earls' mixed field greens salad comes with julienned apples, candied pecans and a generous sprinkle of salty feta cheese. With apple cider vinaigrette, this vitamin-packed salad has just 230 calories. Get the dressing on the side to shave off more calories and cut back the salad's 19 grams of fat.

1 order of Earls Kitchen & Bar warm spinach and feta dip

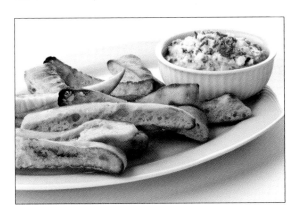

EQUALS

4 1/2 hot dogs

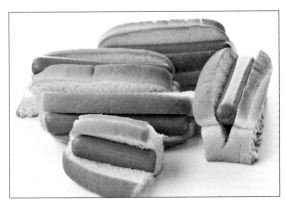

The dip offers up the calorie equivalent of 4 1/2 hot dogs.

JACK ASTOR'S CHEESE GARLIC PAN BREAD

This giant puff of pan bread is a Jack Astor's favourite. It's enjoyed by couples on cozy dates, at the bar with some pints and by hungry families who gobble it up while waiting for their meals.

You may think pan bread isn't much different from the complimentary basket of buns on offer at most restaurants. But the coating of garlic sauce and puddle of cheese at its centre makes Jack's popular pan bread truly calorific. Its dipping sauce—a pot of melted butter—puts it over the edge.

JACK ASTOR'S CHEESE GARLIC PAN BREAD
Calories: 1,179
Fat: 58 grams
Carbohydrates: 128 grams
Protein: 38 grams
Sodium: 1,699
Salt shakes: 42

5 SLICES OF PIZZA
Calories: 1,000
Fat: 35 grams
Carbohydrates: 130 grams
Protein: 50 grams
Sodium: 2,600 mg
Salt shakes: 65

SMART SWAPS: A cup of cheddar cheese soup will satisfy even your cheesiest cravings for 158 calories—the same as what's in about one-eighth of a slice of the pan bread. With 10 grams of fat, the soup is still an indulgent starter. But it is one of the lighter choices among Jack's calorie-laden fare. Or if you love the Cheese Garlic Pan Bread—love it as much as you adored your high school sweetheart—treat it as your main meal by splitting it (preferably in four) and adding on the appetizer house salad. (Tip: the blackberry balsamic dressing gets top nutrition marks.)

1 order of Jack Astor's Cheese Garlic Pan Bread

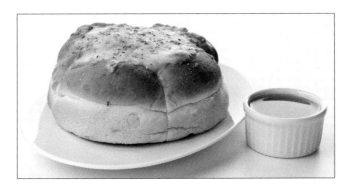

EQUALS

at least 5 slices of pizza

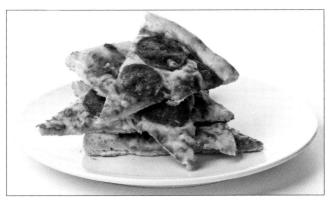

All you really need to know is that this "start-up" has more calories and fat than five pieces of pepperoni pizza.

MOXIE'S CLASSIC GRILL CALAMARI

On most appetizer menus, calamari has replaced shrimp as the go-to seafood starter. That's not necessarily a bad thing. But in the hands of many cooks, plain squid morphs into batter-encrusted, deep-fried, sauce-riddled calamari. Any health benefits get left behind in the fryer.

At Moxie's, crispy rings of calamari are tossed with red onions and served with tzatziki. As expected, this tiny tray contains as many calories as a meal. Like any treat, a few bites would be best.

MOXIE'S CLASSIC GRILL CALAMARI	CHICKEN SOUP Per serving
Calories: 544	Calories: 110
Fat: 39 grams	Fat: 3 grams
Carbohydrates: 23 grams	Carbohydrates: 15 grams
Protein: 25 grams	Protein: 7 grams
Sodium: 583 mg	Sodium: 650 mg
Salt shakes: 14 1/2	Salt shakes: 16

KEY QUESTIONS: Since Moxie's is one of the few Canadian chain restaurants that doesn't post nutrition numbers, it's hard to know which of the appetizers won't sink your meal. This is where questioning your server is important. You might want to ask: Are the avocado spring rolls fried or fresh? Are the pan-seared prawns cooked in butter or heart-healthy olive oil? A few simple questions may save you a few hundred calories.

1 order of Moxie's Classic Grill calamari

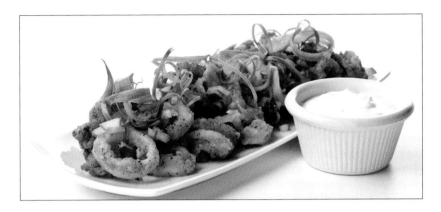

EQUALS

5 servings of chicken soup

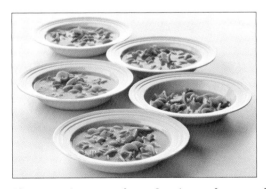

If you eat every ring of calamari, you will have slurped down the calorie and fat equivalent of five servings of store-bought chicken noodle soup.

THE BREAD BASKET

I'm a sucker for the complimentary bread that precedes many restaurant meals. Especially since I usually go to dinner famished. But I know now that nibbling on bread can easily add a few hundred calories to my meal—before the entree arrives—and will negate other good choices I've made. When the server brings the bread basket, I put one large or two small pieces on my side plate if I can't resist. Then I ignore the rest. If the basket bears bread hybrids, like cheese biscuits or greasy corn bread, I leave them untouched. I've learned they are typically no better nutritionally than the doughnuts I dutifully avoid during the day. You might feel the same way, too, after finding out that a pair of cheese biscuits has as many calories and as much fat as two twinkies.

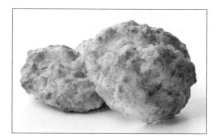

2 Cheddar Bay biscuits at Red Lobster

EQUALS

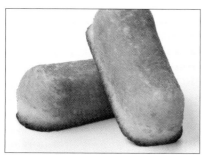

2 twinkies

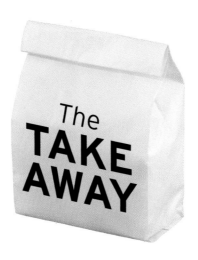

The
TAKE AWAY

Aim for an appetizer centred on fruit or vegetables, whether a mini-plate of greens or a cup of minestrone soup. Fresh, grilled or broiled fish and seafood are also smart choices—but ask your server to make sure the cook omits any added butter or oil.

Be wary of starters that are soaked in sauces or have been through the deep fryer. These are the ones that could pack close to 100 calories per big bite.

Order sauces on the side so you can be in control.

Banish the bread basket if you've ordered an appetizer.

Question the server and ask for substitutes to make the best choice.

Split your favourite appetizer
with your dining companion to divvy up the calories.

Make your favourite appetizer a meal by forgoing the entrees and adding on an appetizer-sized salad.

DINING OUT

It's never been easier to sit down to dinner outside our homes. Familiar chain restaurants can be found in just about every city from coast to coast to coast. Dining out is now an everyday luxury. It's important, then, to make wise choices when selecting from a menu to ensure these frequent outings don't do too much damage to our waistlines.

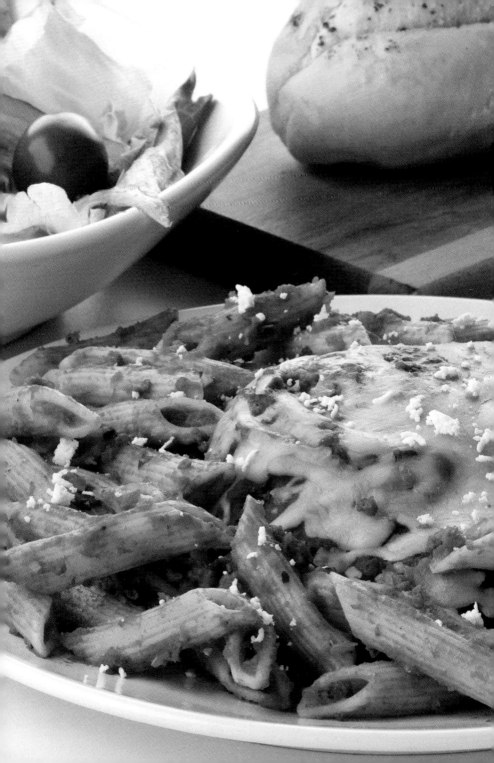

East Side Mario's Classic Chicken Parmigiana with Penne Napolitana

East Side Mario says the classic dishes are the ones that made him famous. Here, Mario's Classic Chicken Parmigiana—a breaded chicken breast, topped with tomato sauce and baked with mozzarella—gets the star turn, accompanied by a side of penne Napolitana.

This meal, already plenty big enough, is preceded by a celebrated opening act: East Side's signature all-you-can-eat soup or salad and garlic homeloaf. People rave about this duo. Some love it more than the main attraction.

We don't know Mario's preferences. But, based on the portion sizes, you can bet he has a very big appetite.

EAST SIDE MARIO'S IDEAL MEAL: If you're looking for the healthiest foods on the East Side, skip over the "classic" entrees and create your own meal from a selection of sides. A cup of minestrone soup, two shrimp skewers paired with pasta (preferably whole wheat) with Napolitana sauce and a side of roasted vegetables has 630 calories, 16 grams of fat and 1,850 mg of sodium. You'll still get a taste of Italy, but you won't be loosening your belt on the way out the door.

DANGER ZONE: Mario cooks up a half-dozen calorie bombs. One of the biggest is the scallop carbonara, which has (without the bread and salad) 1,390 calories and 78 grams of fat—more fat than what's found in five orders of onion rings at Harvey's.

EAST SIDE MARIO'S
CLASSIC CHICKEN
PARMIGIANA WITH PENNE
NAPOLITANA

GARDEN SALAD,
SINGLE SERVING
Calories: 190
Fat: 15 grams
Carbohydrates: 10 grams
Protein: 2 grams
Sodium: 680 mg
Salt shakes: 17

GARLIC HOMELOAF
Calories: 300
Fat: 7 grams
Carbohydrates: 49 grams
Protein: 9 grams
Sodium: 650 mg
Salt shakes: 16

CHICKEN PARMIGIANA
Calories: 500
Fat: 14 grams
Carbohydrates: 42 grams
Protein: 41 grams
Sodium: 1,890 mg
Salt shakes: 47

PENNE WITH NAPOLITANA
SAUCE
Calories: 370
Fat: 8 grams
Carbohydrates: 63 grams
Protein: 11 grams
Sodium: 850 mg
Salt shakes: 21

ICED TEA, 355 ML
Calories: 120
Carbohydrates: 34 grams

TOTAL
Calories: 1,480
Fat: 44 grams
Carbohydrates: 198 grams
Protein: 63 grams
Sodium: 4,070 mg
Salt shakes: 101

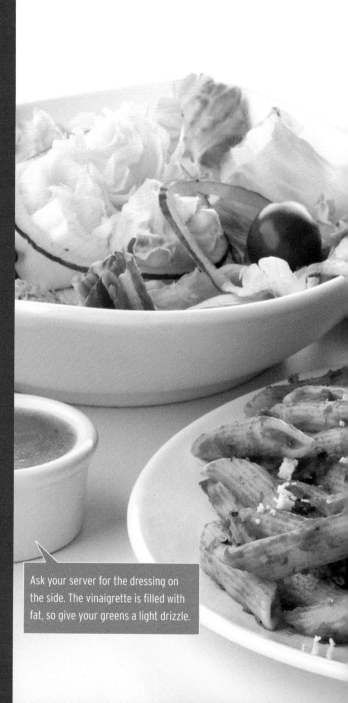

Ask your server for the dressing on
the side. The vinaigrette is filled with
fat, so give your greens a light drizzle.

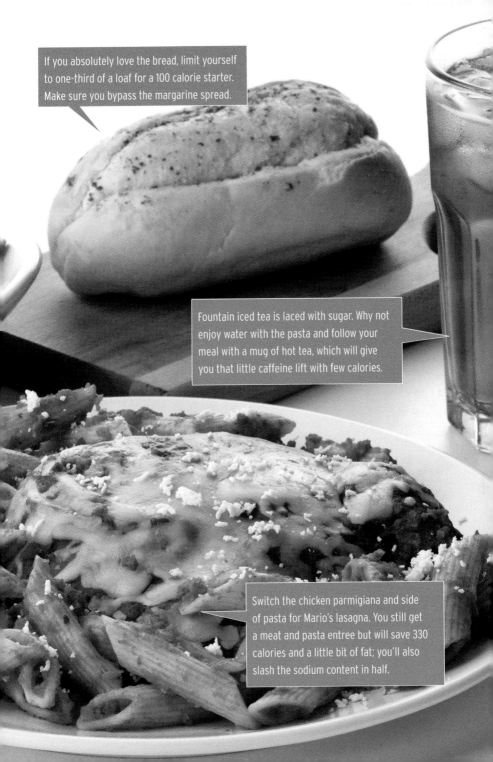

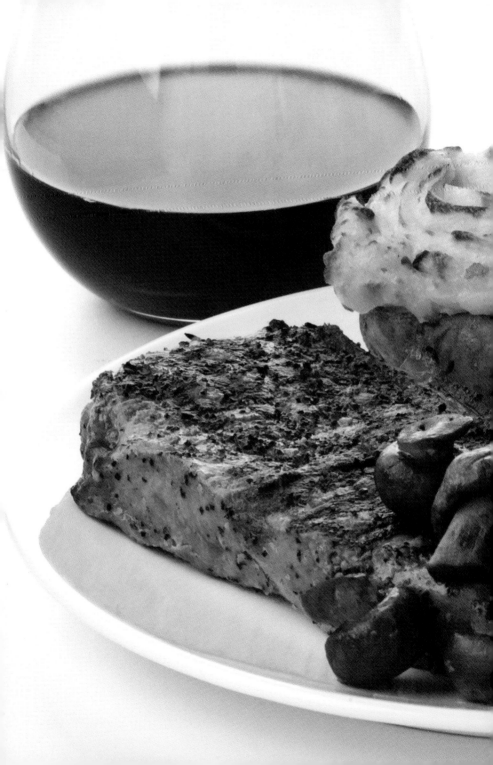

The Keg New York Classic Dinner

The Keg has perfected steakhouse chic. Cloth napkins. Embossed menus. White-aproned servers who proffer plates with a smile and pleasant nod.

The Keg's Classic Dinners are perennial favourites. Diners get a salad, a steak and a serving of vegetables and sautéed mushrooms. Those who can't eat meat without a spud add a potato to their meal.

With the right picks and portion sizes, a Keg Classic Dinner can be decadent but not diet busting. It can also be a calorie disaster—especially if you complete your steakhouse experience with a dessert.

THE KEG'S IDEAL MEAL: The Sirloin Classic Dinner is one of the best choices at The Keg. Skip the potato (you have to pay extra for it, anyway), get the Caesar salad with half the dressing and, with a glass of red wine, you have an elegant and ample meal for 750 calories and 31 grams of fat. While the numbers are still higher than what's recommended for a meal, many other Keg meals can have triple those calories.

DANGER ZONE: The dessert menu is deadly. Of the six full-sized items, three have more than 800 calories and 40 grams of fat. That's like finishing your meal with two bacon cheeseburgers from McDonald's! Steer clear, way, way clear, of the crème brûlée, the chocolate cake and the brownie sundae.

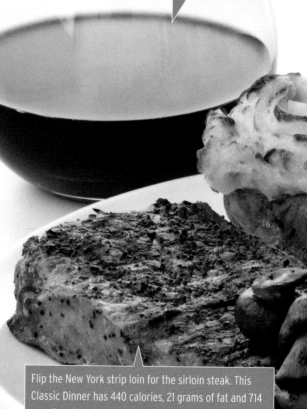

THE KEG NEW YORK CLASSIC DINNER

RED WINE,
6 OUNCE (175 ML)
Calories: 150
Carbohydrates: 5 grams

CAESAR SALAD
Calories: 289
Fat: 20 grams
Carbohydrates: 22 grams
Protein: 7 grams
Sodium: 775 mg
Salt shakes: 19

12-OUNCE NEW YORK
STRIP LOIN STEAK,
WITH VEGETABLES AND
MUSHROOMS
Calories: 753
Fat: 46 grams
Carbohydrates: 11 grams
Protein: 74 grams
Sodium: 934 mg
Salt shakes: 23

TWICE-BAKED POTATO
Calories: 385
Fat: 10 grams
Carbohydrates: 61 grams
Protein: 13 grams
Sodium: 570 mg
Salt shakes: 14

TOTAL
Calories: 1,577
Fat: 76 grams
Carbohydrates: 99 grams
Protein: 94 grams
Sodium: 2,279 mg
Salt shakes: 57

Research has shown that drinking a moderate amount of alcohol protects against heart disease. And red wine, with its plethora of antioxidants, seems to have more heart-healthy benefits than other alcoholic drinks.

Flip the New York strip loin for the sirloin steak. This Classic Dinner has 440 calories, 21 grams of fat and 714 mg of sodium. The difference in numbers may be due to portion size—the sirloin weighs 4 ounces less—but sirloin is one of the leanest cuts of beef.

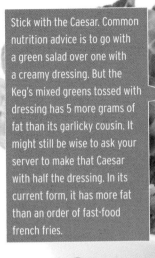

Stick with the Caesar. Common nutrition advice is to go with a green salad over one with a creamy dressing. But the Keg's mixed greens tossed with dressing has 5 more grams of fat than its garlicky cousin. It might still be wise to ask your server to make that Caesar with half the dressing. In its current form, it has more fat than an order of fast-food french fries.

Can you manage without a starch? A double order of classic vegetables adds just 55 calories to the meal.

To cut the fat in your spud, order a potato that has been baked only once. A fluffy baked potato straight from the oven has zero fat. Top it with salsa or a smidgen of sour cream. Beware the roasted-garlic mashed potatoes. This side has more than twice the fat of the twice-baked potato.

This meal has more than three-quarters of your daily calorie needs. If you're a woman, it has 10 more grams of fat than the average recommended daily allotment. (Men, it's just a little bit shy of your daily fat needs.) It also has 50% more sodium than your body needs in a day.

A restaurant critic weighs in

Amy Pataki, the *Toronto Star*'s restaurant critic, has been reviewing restaurants since 2001. At least three times a week she's on the job, nibbling appetizers and tasting entrees at some of Toronto's newest and neatest establishments. While she reveals little about her appearance to maintain her anonymity, it's safe to say Amy is not carrying around 10 years of calories from her professional ventures into restaurants.

You dine out for a living. Do you ever get tired of looking at menus, or do you still get excited about a meal out?
I love going out to eat, anywhere and any time—except for my birthday. That's when I want home-cooked food.

What are the main things you consider for your reviews? Is nutrition ever part of your critique?
I rate restaurants based on the food, service and ambience. Nutrition doesn't figure into it, even when I'm writing about a triple-bacon cheeseburger. Is it a good triple-bacon cheeseburger? Did they bring it quickly, with a smile? Am I eating on a vintage Pac-Man console? I put that information in the review and let readers make the choice.

Do you see a trend towards lighter, healthier fare?
What I see more of in restaurants are unstructured menus where traditional appetizer and main-course categories are replaced with small plates, such as tapas. The trick is to not order too many.

I'm grateful that our restaurants haven't taken to serving large, American-sized portions.

When you're dining out for work, you can't avoid the foie gras or the creamy pasta dishes or the decadent custard desserts. So how do you stay so slim?

Ha! The only way to stay healthy in this job is to exercise. I exercise five days a week for at least 30 minutes a session. Strength training, brisk walking, yoga, belly dancing, biking, personal trainers, the whole bit. I also recently took up running. My fortysomething knees don't love it, but my waistline does.

When you began your career, were you ever worried that dining out so much would affect your health?

I got a baseline level on my cholesterol to see if that would change. So far, it's normal.

What do you worry most about: calories, fat or sodium?

Fat, especially since it's hidden in restaurant meals. Who knows how much butter or oil went into the skillet? Or onto the vegetables.

What strategies have you picked up over the years?

Never clean your plate. Drink water. Split dessert. When I'm eating out on my own time, I skip the appetizer. Or I order two appetizers and skip the main.

When you're going out to eat with family or friends, and you've left the notebook at home, what kinds of restaurants do you find yourself going to over and over again?

Places with intelligent service. Places where my children are welcome. Places without throbbing music. Places that do one type of dish extremely well, like pizza, kebabs, noodle soup or sushi. Nowhere formal.

And yes, we eat at McDonald's once a month, at least. I order a Big Mac and a small Diet Coke but no fries: there are enough fries left over from my three children's Happy Meals to satisfy that craving.

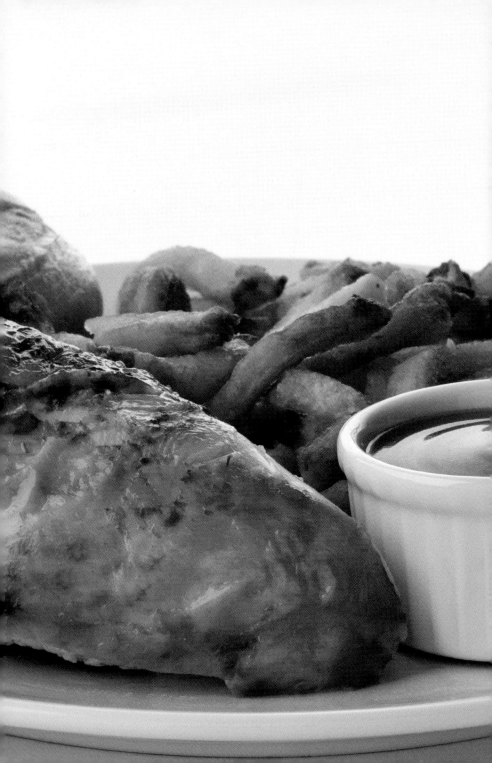

Swiss Chalet Quarter Chicken Dinner

For many of us, Swiss Chalet is the ultimate comfort food. Especially on cold, wintery Canadian nights.

You know a meal is popular when diners don't need to crack the menu. Most already know, before pushing open the Chalet's door, that they will be ordering a Quarter Chicken Dinner.

DANGER ZONE: There aren't too many calorie conundrums at Swiss Chalet. But the rather harmless-sounding rotisserie chicken club wrap has 710 calories and 32 grams of fat. Without a side! Calorie-wise, that's like eating two orders of chicken strips from Harvey's.

SWISS CHALET'S IDEAL MEAL: It's easy to find. The Heart and Stroke Foundation's Health Check program identifies meals that have adequate amounts of protein, two servings of fruits or vegetables and limited amounts of fat and sodium. One of these meals is the Chalet's chicken on a kaiser roll. With sweet kernel corn (and no Chalet dipping sauce), this meal has 630 calories, 14 grams of fat and 960 mg of sodium.

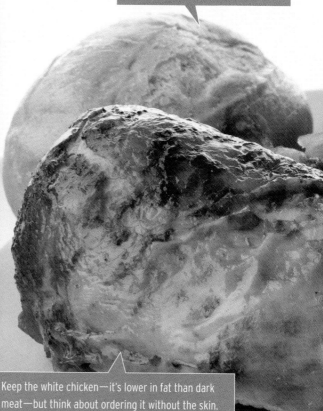

SWISS CHALET QUARTER CHICKEN DINNER

WHITE ROLL
Calories: 110
Fat: 0 grams
Carbohydrates: 22 grams
Protein: 4 grams
Sodium: 190 mg
Salt shakes: 5

QUARTER CHICKEN, WHITE MEAT WITH SKIN
Calories: 290
Fat: 11 grams
Carbohydrates: 0 grams
Protein: 48 grams
Sodium: 330 mg
Salt shakes: 8

FRENCH FRIES
Calories: 530
Fat: 27 grams
Carbohydrates: 64 grams
Protein: 7 grams
Sodium: 95 mg
Salt shakes: 2

CHALET DIPPING SAUCE
Calories: 25
Fat: 0.5 grams
Carbohydrates: 5 grams
Protein: 0 grams
Sodium: 700 mg
Salt shakes: 17 1/2

TOTAL
Calories: 955
Fat: 38.5 grams
Carbohydrates: 91 grams
Protein: 59 grams
Sodium: 1,315 mg
Salt shakes: 32 1/2

With the fries, the Quarter Chicken Dinner has half your daily calories and fat. And it's just 200 mg shy of your sodium needs for the day.

Pick multigrain bread over white whenever you can. The choice may not impact calories, but it will provide nutritional benefits.

Keep the white chicken—it's lower in fat than dark meat—but think about ordering it without the skin. Peeling it off will save 70 calories and 5 grams of fat.

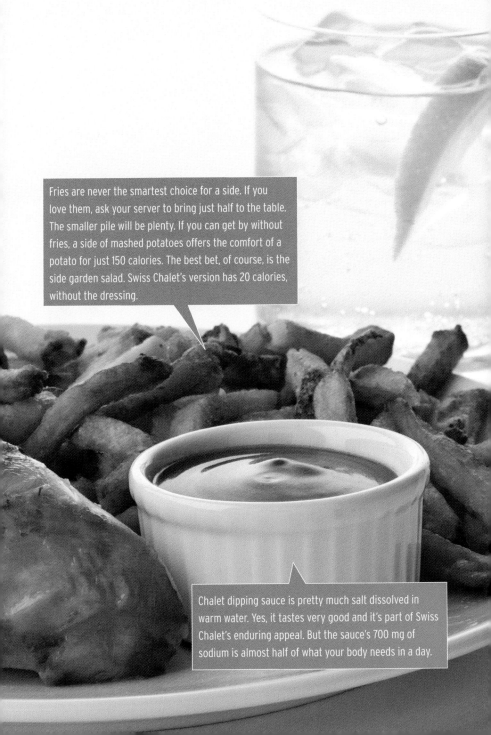

Fries are never the smartest choice for a side. If you love them, ask your server to bring just half to the table. The smaller pile will be plenty. If you can get by without fries, a side of mashed potatoes offers the comfort of a potato for just 150 calories. The best bet, of course, is the side garden salad. Swiss Chalet's version has 20 calories, without the dressing.

Chalet dipping sauce is pretty much salt dissolved in warm water. Yes, it tastes very good and it's part of Swiss Chalet's enduring appeal. But the sauce's 700 mg of sodium is almost half of what your body needs in a day.

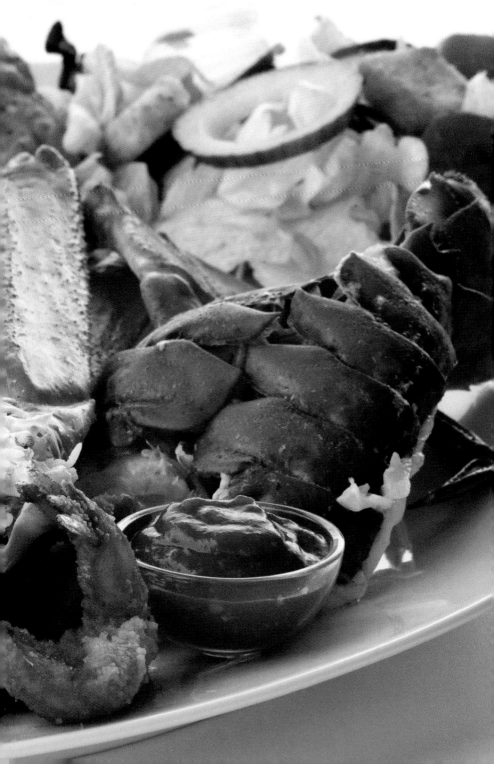

Red Lobster Ultimate Feast

Forgo the fryer at Red Lobster and it's hard to pile thousands of calories on your plate. Even the Ultimate Feast—a moniker that would usually raise a red flag—won't be *that* detrimental to your waistline. But only if you make a few substitutions. Make no changes and the Ultimate Feast is an ultimate disaster. It has more than half your daily calories, more than two-thirds of your fat allowance and *twice* the maximum daily sodium recommendation. That's like dumping 2 rounded teaspoons of salt over your meal.

DANGER ZONE: Avoid the seafood starters and stick to Red Lobster's main menu, where it's easier to make a right step than a wrong one. Even if you tread carefully among the appetizers, you are bound to go under. The Crispy Calamari and Vegetables has 97 grams of fat—the amount a man should consume in a day. The Lobster-Artichoke-and-Seafood Dip is just as scary. It has the same amount of fat as 37 Honey Dip Timbits.

RED LOBSTER'S IDEAL MEAL: Your best bet at Red Lobster, nutrition-wise, is to order a piece of grilled, broiled or blackened fresh fish with lots of vegetable sides.

RED LOBSTER ULTIMATE FEAST

2 CHEDDAR BAY BISCUITS
Calories: 300
Fat: 16 grams
Carbohydrates: 32 grams
Protein: 6 grams
Sodium: 700 mg
Salt shakes: 17 1/2

GARLIC-GRILLED SHRIMP
Calories: 60
Fat: 1 gram
Carbohydrates: 0 grams
Protein: 12 grams
Sodium: 580 mg
Salt shakes: 14 1/2

GARDEN SALAD WITH BALSAMIC DRESSING
Calories: 170
Fat: 9 grams
Carbohydrates: 17 grams
Protein: 2 grams
Sodium: 295 mg
Salt shakes: 7

WALT'S FAVOURITE SHRIMP
Calories: 370
Fat: 20 grams
Carbohydrates: 25 grams
Protein: 21 grams
Sodium: 1,500 mg
Salt shakes: 37 1/2

LOBSTER TAIL
Calories: 60
Fat: 0.5 grams
Carbohydrates: 0 grams
Protein: 14 grams
Sodium: 490 mg
Salt shakes: 12

MASHED POTATOES
Calories: 210
Fat: 10 grams
Carbohydrates: 27 grams
Protein: 5 grams
Sodium: 620 mg
Salt shakes: 15 1/2

SNOW CRAB LEGS (1/2 POUND)
Calories: 90
Fat: 1 gram
Carbohydrates: 0 grams
Protein: 20 grams
Sodium: 790 mg
Salt shakes: 20

TOTAL
Calories: 1,260
Fat: 57.5 grams
Carbohydrates: 101 grams
Protein: 80 grams
Sodium: 4,975 mg
Salt shakes: 124

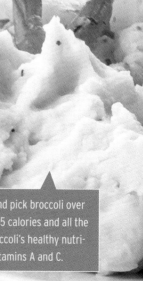

The sodium in the seafood is astronomical. But if you look strictly at calories and fat, the numbers are impressively low for such a big plate. With the double order of garlic-grilled shrimp, all this seafood has 270 calories and less than 4 grams of fat.

Add more colour to the plate and pick broccoli over mashed potatoes. You'll save 165 calories and all the fat, plus get the benefits of broccoli's healthy nutrients, including folic acid and vitamins A and C.

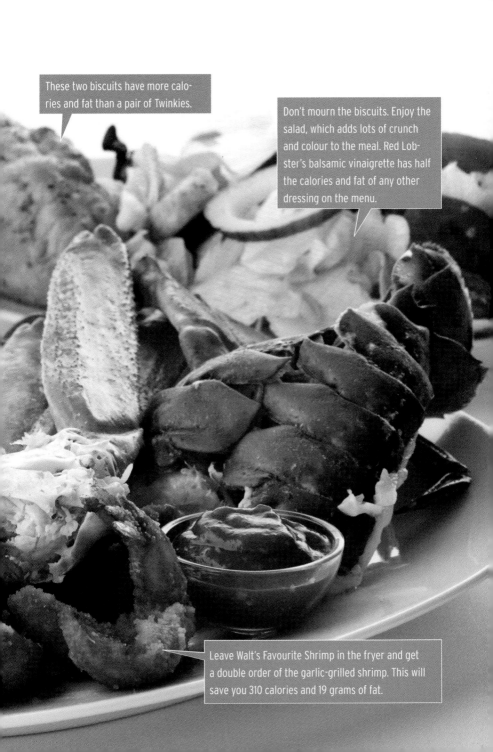

These two biscuits have more calories and fat than a pair of Twinkies.

Don't mourn the biscuits. Enjoy the salad, which adds lots of crunch and colour to the meal. Red Lobster's balsamic vinaigrette has half the calories and fat of any other dressing on the menu.

Leave Walt's Favourite Shrimp in the fryer and get a double order of the garlic-grilled shrimp. This will save you 310 calories and 19 grams of fat.

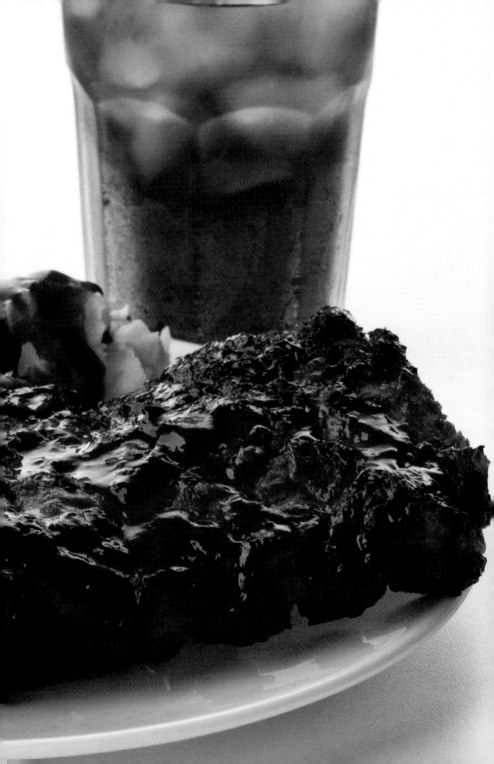

Montana's Cookhouse Smokehouse Pork Back Ribs

The folks at Montana's encourage meat lovers to escape to the Cookhouse, where plenty of carnivorous fare fills the menu. You can choose from pork back ribs, roast chicken, sizzling steaks and fat, juicy burgers. Yes, many of these meaty mains are calorific. But it's the sides that can turn a hefty plate into a meal that only a worn-out cowboy—one who has just spent 14 hours in the mountains wrangling cattle—should ever eat.

DANGER ZONE: Montana's Smokehouse Wrap, made with pulled chicken, chopped bacon, rice, tomatoes, green onion and grated cheese is drizzled with barbeque sauce and Caesar dressing. On its own, this wrap has more than half your daily calories and three-quarters of your day's fat. Without a side.

MONTANA'S IDEAL MEAL: With some omissions and a swap, this meal could be one of the Cookhouse's better choices. Without the cornbread and gravy, and substituting the sirloin for the ribs, this platter has 520 calories, 20 grams of fat and 1,050 mg of sodium. That's two-thirds fewer calories, two-thirds less fat and two-thirds less sodium.

MONTANA'S COOK-HOUSE SMOKEHOUSE PORK BACK RIBS

COOKHOUSE CORNBREAD, 1 PIECE
Calories: 260
Fat: 11 grams
Carbohydrates: 39 grams
Protein: 4 grams
Sodium: 330 mg
Salt shakes: 8

PORK BACK RIBS, REGULAR SIZE
Calories: 870
Fat: 58 grams
Carbohydrates: 41 grams
Protein: 45 grams
Sodium: 1,380 mg
Salt shakes: 34 1/2

MASHED POTATOES
Calories: 110
Fat: 3 grams
Carbohydrates: 19 grams
Protein: 2 grams
Sodium: 350 mg
Salt shakes: 9

GRAVY
Calories: 25
Fat: 4 grams
Carbohydrates: 5 grams
Protein: 1 gram
Sodium: 440 mg
Salt shakes: 11

COLESLAW
Calories: 80
Fat: 5 grams
Carbohydrates: 7 grams
Protein: 1 gram
Sodium: 240 mg
Salt shakes: 6

COKE, 355 ML
Calories: 140
Carbohydrates: 42 grams

TOTAL
Calories: 1,485
Fat: 77.5 grams
Carbohydrates: 153 grams
Protein: 53 grams
Sodium: 2,740 mg
Salt shakes: 68 1/2

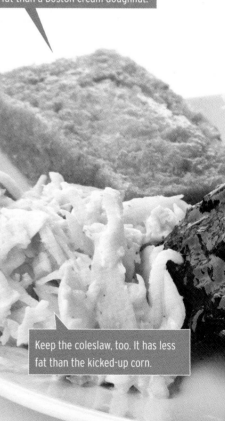

Chuck the cornbread under the wagon. It has more calories and fat than a Boston cream doughnut.

Keep the coleslaw, too. It has less fat than the kicked-up corn.

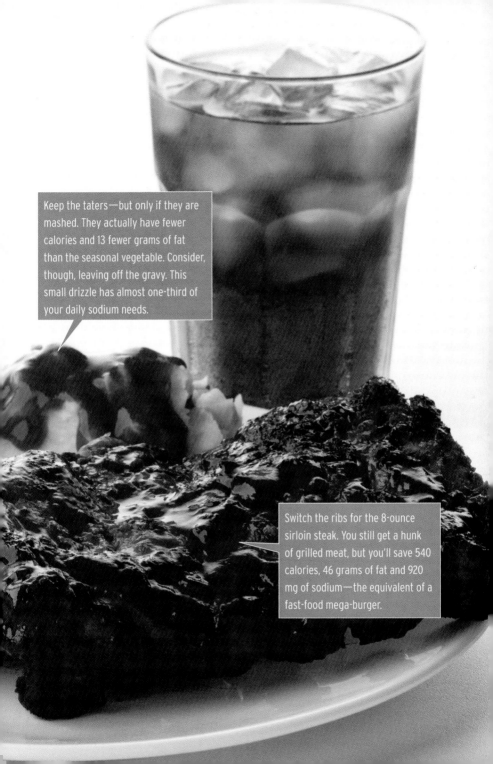

Keep the taters—but only if they are mashed. They actually have fewer calories and 13 fewer grams of fat than the seasonal vegetable. Consider, though, leaving off the gravy. This small drizzle has almost one-third of your daily sodium needs.

Switch the ribs for the 8-ounce sirloin steak. You still get a hunk of grilled meat, but you'll save 540 calories, 46 grams of fat and 920 mg of sodium—the equivalent of a fast-food mega-burger.

Dining out with a dietitian

Carol Harrison has been a registered dietitian for 20 years. The busy mom of three believes the only food worth eating is food that tastes terrific. She also believes that terrific-tasting food can indeed be healthy.

Carol finds it easy to follow her eating philosophy at home, where she whips up meals and snacks for her family. But when Carol dines out—which is once every week or two—it can be harder to find a meal that tickles her taste buds and satisfies her inner dietitian. One way Carol finds that balance when eating outside her home is to decide ahead of time whether the meal is a treat or simply fuel to power her through the remainder of the day. If it's an indulgence—for Carol that means food that is authentic and made with wholesome, seasonal ingredients—then she enjoys every bite. If she is popping into a chain restaurant for a quick meal, then Carol sticks to her dietitian training, putting health ahead of taste.

Carol says she hopes one day soon Canadian restaurants will see that diners want the same thing she does—healthy, wholesome foods that taste terrific—and make these the go-to choices on menus, rather than the exception. And, she adds, diners can help push restaurants by asking for healthier choices each time they dine out. "Try ordering brown rice instead of white at your favourite Chinese restaurant, or requesting more vegetables in your chicken pad Thai," she says. "If we ask for these healthy choices enough, the industry will respond."

Carol's top tips for dining out

- Enjoy your food—always.
- If you eat out often, say, more than one or two times a week, search out better choices. Look for meals made with whole grains, vegetables, lean meats, beans or eggs, and dishes with little or no added fat. You might be surprised by how great they taste. And your waistline will thank you.
- Ask to see the nutrition information or do some online investigating before you head to the restaurant. Nutrition land mines can be all over the menu, and what you think might be a good choice could be a great big salt lick! Once you know what the better choices are, you don't need to keep checking.
- Ask questions. Find out how the food is made—what's in it and how it is cooked and if there are any healthier trades you can make.
- Ask for what you want. Restaurants want satisfied customers.
- If you do only one thing to make dining out a healthy experience, let it be this: Expect big portions and eat half. "That's the single best piece of advice I can give," says Carol.

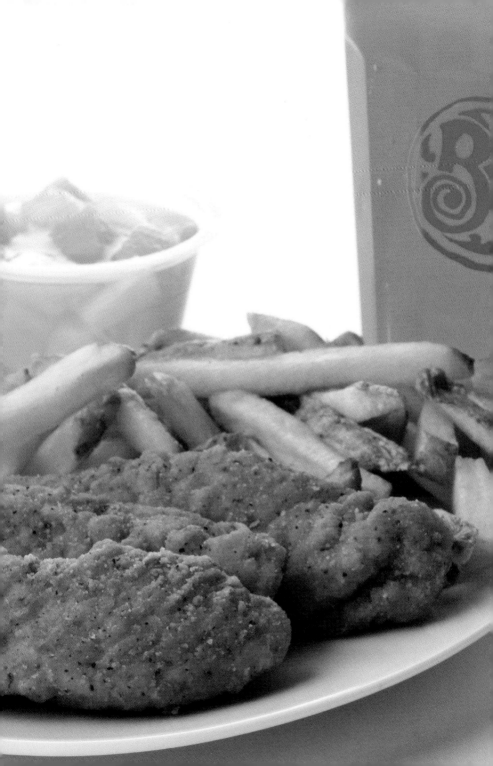

Boston Pizza chicken fingers (kids' meal)

Boston Pizza may be known for its pizza. But according to an informal survey of servers, most patrons under the age of 10 go for the plate of chicken fingers with fries. This family-friendly restaurant offers its youngest diners a choice of seven entrees with a choice of side, dessert and activity book. Along with the typical kiddie standards of pizza and cheesy noodles there is also some grown-up (and healthier) fare.

DANGER ZONE: We all know the dessert menu can be deadly. But would you guess that the pint-sized sundae, meant for a kid under the age of 10, would have 480 calories and 22 grams of fat? This "small" treat is equivalent, both calorie- and fat-wise, to 10 chocolate sandwich cookies. The Worms & Dirt—that's chocolate pudding with gummy worms—has an incredible 420 calories and 13 grams of fat.

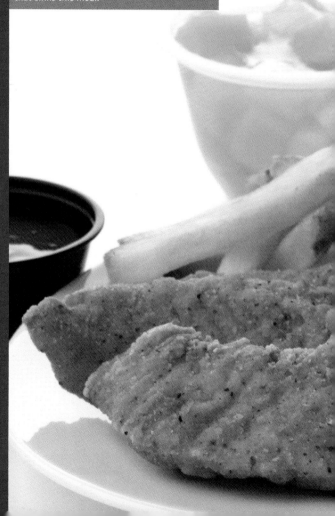

BOSTON PIZZA CHICKEN FINGERS (KIDS' MEAL)

CHICKEN FINGERS
Calories: 250
Fat: 10 grams
Carbohydrates: 29 grams
Protein: 14 grams
Sodium: 640 mg
Salt shakes: 16

FRENCH FRIES
Calories: 180 calories
Fat: 7 grams
Carbohydrates: 27 grams
Protein: 2 grams
Sodium: 630 mg
Salt shakes: 16

ORANGE SODA, 250 ML
Calories: 125
Carbohydrates: 37 grams

FRUIT CUP
Calories: 80
Fat: 0 grams
Carbohydrates: 19 grams
Protein: 0 grams
Sodium: 0 mg
Salt shakes: 0

TOTAL
Calories: 635
Fat: 17 grams
Carbohydrates: 112 grams
Protein: 16 grams
Sodium: 1,270 mg
Salt shakes: 32

Your child's dietary needs will be different depending on his age, height, weight and activity level. But for the average nine-year-old boy, this meal contains about one-third of his calories, about 40% of his daily 44 grams of fat and 85% of his sodium. It's the saltiness that sinks this meal.

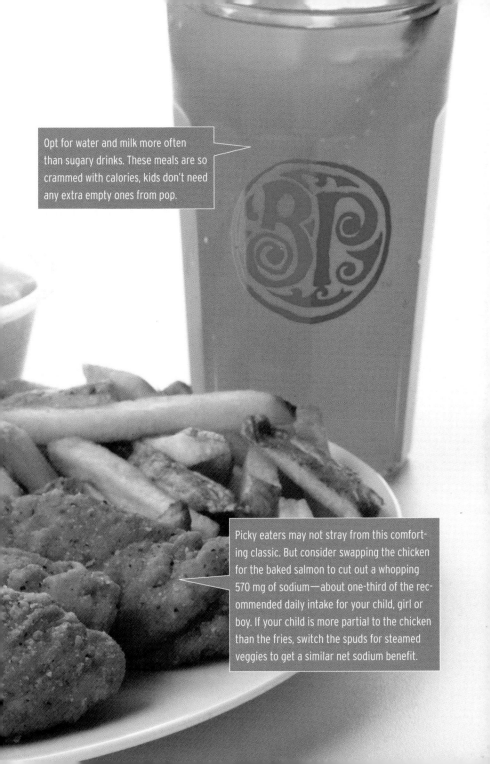

Opt for water and milk more often than sugary drinks. These meals are so crammed with calories, kids don't need any extra empty ones from pop.

Picky eaters may not stray from this comforting classic. But consider swapping the chicken for the baked salmon to cut out a whopping 570 mg of sodium—about one-third of the recommended daily intake for your child, girl or boy. If your child is more partial to the chicken than the fries, switch the spuds for steamed veggies to get a similar net sodium benefit.

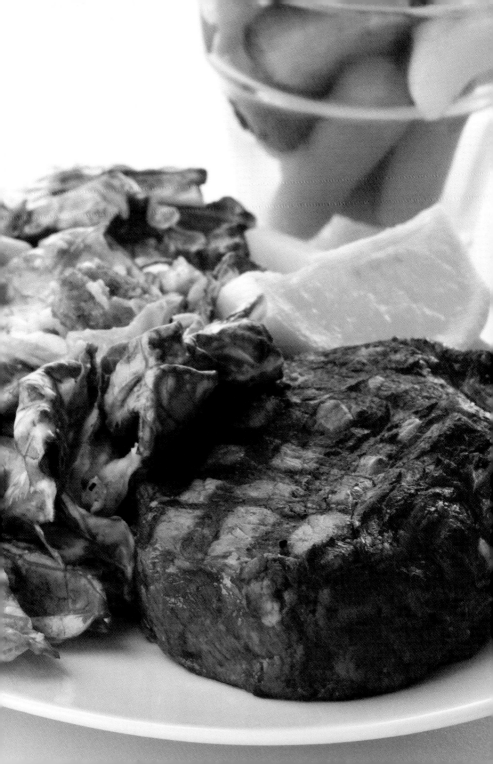

The Keg Kid's Sirloin Dinner

For kids, the cool thing about eating at The Keg is that the child-sized meal looks a lot like the one Mom and Dad might get—except that it has milk instead of wine.

Kids get veggies as an appetizer, a steak, and the choice of fries, seasonal vegetables or the classic Caesar salad. They also get a drink—pop, juice or milk—and ice cream for dessert. They will feel very grown up.

DANGER ZONE: The "kid's" ice cream is the killer here. Take out the dessert and this meal has 679 calories and 33 grams of fat and 225 mg less sodium. If you must keep it, get several spoons. For the average 13-year-old girl, this meal (without dessert) has about one-third of her daily calories and 60% of her day's worth of fat. The 1,499 mg of sodium—the most worrisome thing about the meal—takes up all of her daily sodium requirements.

THE KEG KIDS' SIRLOIN DINNER

6-OUNCE KID'S SIRLOIN
Calories: 244
Fat: 11 grams
Carbohydrates: 0 grams
Protein: 37 grams
Sodium: 559 mg
Salt shakes: 14

VEGETABLES WITH RANCH DRESSING
Calories: 170
Fat: 10 grams
Carbohydrates: 20 grams
Protein: 2 grams
Sodium: 418 mg
Salt shakes: 11

CAESAR SALAD (HALF-PORTION OF ADULT SERVING)
Calories: 145
Fat: 10 grams
Carbohydrates: 11 grams
Protein: 4 grams
Sodium: 388 mg
Salt shakes: 10

MILK, 1%, 250 ML
Calories: 112
Fat: 2.5 grams
Carbohydrates: 13 grams
Protein: 9 grams
Sodium: 135 mg
Salt shakes: 3

KID'S ICE CREAM
Calories: 473
Fat: 24 grams
Carbohydrates: 62 grams
Protein: 5 grams
Sodium: 225 mg
Salt shakes: 6

TOTAL
Calories: 1,152
Fat: 57.5 grams
Carbohydrates: 106 grams
Protein: 57 grams
Sodium: 1,725 mg
Salt shakes: 43

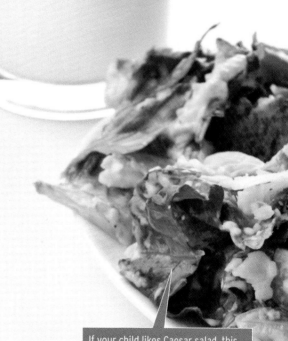

About one-third of kids don't get enough servings of dairy products a day. Keep the milk to make sure your child gets her calcium quota.

If your child likes Caesar salad, this is a good way for her to get her greens. At the Keg, the Caesar is a better bet than fries.

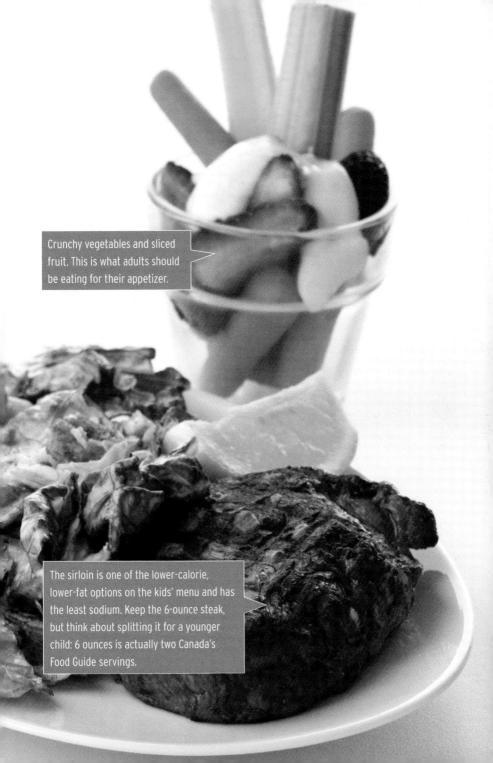

Crunchy vegetables and sliced fruit. This is what adults should be eating for their appetizer.

The sirloin is one of the lower-calorie, lower-fat options on the kids' menu and has the least sodium. Keep the 6-ounce steak, but think about splitting it for a younger child: 6 ounces is actually two Canada's Food Guide servings.

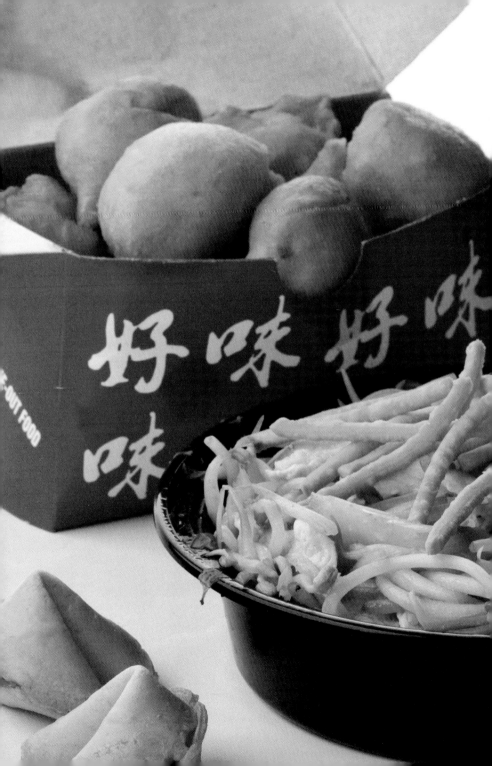

The Mandarin
Special Family Dinner for Two

The Mandarin is famous for its seemingly endless all-you-can-eat buffet. Soups, salads, breads, rice dishes, noodle dishes, chicken dishes, fresh-carved roast beef, potatoes, vegetables, steamed buns, sushi, ice cream, cakes, custards . . . it's a glut of food.

Its takeout menu offers just a fraction of the selection. But the portions stuffed into the takeout containers will leave you just as full as if you'd navigated the buffet.

SMART SWAP: In this Dinner for Two, a set meal on the takeout menu, much of the fare is fried. Ordering off the à la carte menu will give you more selection and help pare back the overload of calories. For example, consider ordering the chicken with almonds and vegetables instead of the fried sweet-and-sour chicken balls. The breaded pieces of chicken contain about 115 calories each.

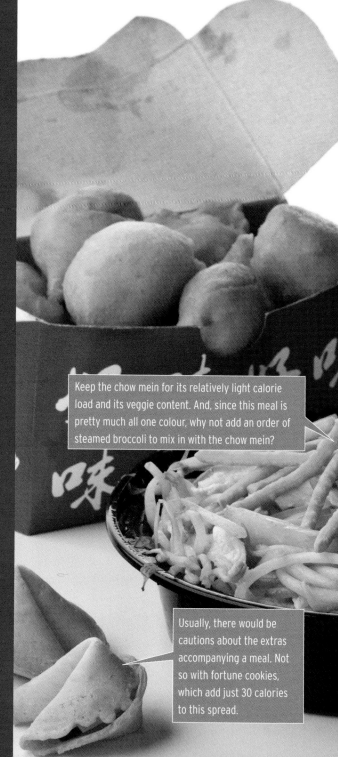

THE MANDARIN SPECIAL FAMILY DINNER FOR TWO

2 EGG ROLLS
Calories: 263
Fat: 14 grams
Carbohydrates: 25 grams
Protein: 8 grams
Sodium: 335 mg
Salt shakes: 8

CHICKEN BALLS
Calories: 1,131
Fat: 50 grams
Carbohydrates: 118 grams
Protein: 53 grams
Sodium: 1,547 mg
Salt shakes: 39

CHICKEN FRIED RICE
Calories: 1,172
Fat: 15 grams
Carbohydrates: 176 grams
Protein: 85 grams
Sodium: 2,374 mg
Salt shakes: 59

CHICKEN CHOW MEIN
Calories: 667
Fat: 28 grams
Carbohydrates: 32 grams
Protein: 71 grams
Sodium: 1,723 mg
Salt shakes: 43

TOTAL PER PERSON
Calories: 1,616
Fat: 53 grams
Carbohydrates: 175 grams
Protein: 108 grams
Sodium: 2,989 mg
Salt shakes: 75

Keep the chow mein for its relatively light calorie load and its veggie content. And, since this meal is pretty much all one colour, why not add an order of steamed broccoli to mix in with the chow mein?

Usually, there would be cautions about the extras accompanying a meal. Not so with fortune cookies, which add just 30 calories to this spread.

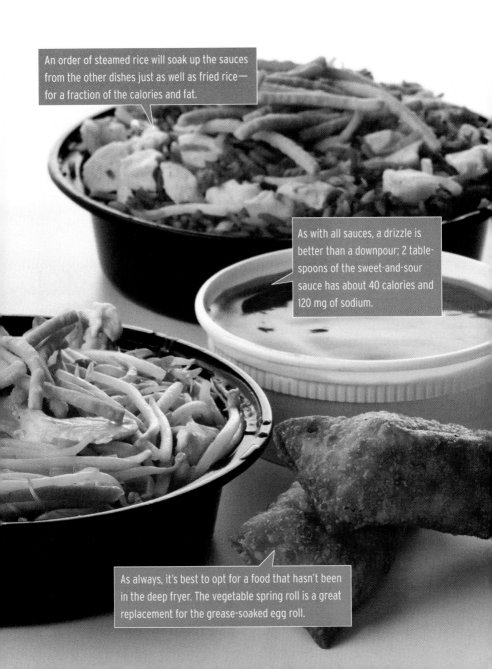

For the average woman, splitting this meal gives her 80% of her day's calories and fat and two times her daily sodium requirements.

An order of steamed rice will soak up the sauces from the other dishes just as well as fried rice— for a fraction of the calories and fat.

As with all sauces, a drizzle is better than a downpour; 2 table-spoons of the sweet-and-sour sauce has about 40 calories and 120 mg of sodium.

As always, it's best to opt for a food that hasn't been in the deep fryer. The vegetable spring roll is a great replacement for the grease-soaked egg roll.

How to negotiate kids' menus

Zannat Reza, a registered dietitian with 14 years of experience, considers dining out with her family a treat. Her two young children cheerily chomp on carrot and celery sticks but are also known to dig into a pile of french fries. For a class snack they might take strawberries—which go over with their friends surprisingly well. Zannat's favourite foods are chocolate, mango and guava. Her mantra is that good-for-you foods have to taste great.

How does Zannat, the dietitian, react to the typical kids' menus? How does Zannat, the parent, react?
The dietitian and the parent react in the same way—I'm not crazy about kids' menus generally. Because we eat out as a treat, I don't mind too much if they choose a less-than-healthy option. After all, it's one meal out of the whole week or month, and we tend to eat pretty well most of the time.

How do you negotiate the multi-course kids' meals?
By making the best choices we can in each course. We ask for less, or split them. We usually order chocolate milk or 100% juice as the beverage. Some kids' meals are still too big for kids. It's always possible to take some of the meal home or to skip the dessert.

What if you skip the kids' menu entirely?
Splitting an entree off the regular menu is a great way to eat better. You can also order a couple of healthier sides to make a meal, such as a baked potato, chicken or shrimp skewers and steamed veggies. My kids love salmon, chicken and steak. We went to a Colombian restaurant recently, and I split my chicken fajitas with them—the portion was huge, so it was great for sharing. They loved it!

Are there one or two items you can always count on to be healthier choices for your kids?
A small cheese pizza, pasta with tomato sauce or a small burger.

How about kid-food catastrophes—dishes that are best to avoid?
Hot dogs are a definite no-no. They are highly processed, high in salt and usually full of preservatives.

Should parents also pay attention to sodium on behalf of their kids?
More and more kids are developing high blood pressure, something that we can't see. Restaurant foods tend to be high in salt, so I do think parents need to be aware of what they're allowing their kids to eat. Trying to get a balance of vegetables and fruit, whole grains, milk and lean protein is key to fuelling your kids the right way.

Do you and your kids make different choices if you dine out once a month compared with sitting down at a restaurant once or twice a week?
Because we don't dine out a whole lot, the kids can get french fries if they want. Fries are something they don't get at home—though I bake my own sweet potato fries. After all, dining out needs to be a pleasant experience, and not one that turns into a food fight. If we ate out more often, then I would put down more boundaries.

Is it important for kids to see their parents passing on french fries?
Parents are role models. Kids watch our choices very carefully. So either pass on the fries or split them and order a veggie plate to share for the table. The kids may complain, but over time it gets ingrained.

What's the biggest nutrition struggle in your family while dining out? How do you resolve it?

Finding vegetables and fruit that the kids will like and eat. Overcooked veggies are a big turnoff. And some raw veggies are hard for young kids to eat. If a restaurant meal is low in fruit and vegetables, we make it up at the next meal or snack.

Zannat's top tips for dining out with kids

- If possible, scope out the kids' menu online. Set any ground rules before you go so you're not dealing with a tantrum once the kids realize you're setting boundaries.
- Choose a meal from the regular menu and split it with your child or between your kids. Try grilled chicken, pasta with tomato sauce and meatballs, a colourful stir-fry or grilled salmon.
- Order a healthier appetizer as a main course for your child—for example, chicken skewers, fresh spring rolls or quesadillas.
- If your kids have already had a treat that day, let them know that's why they won't be having a sugary dessert.
- Order fresh fruit as a side. That way, your kids will have less space for dessert.
- If fries are too much of a battle, ask for fewer fries on the plate, share them with the whole table, or order half fries, half veggies. Sweet potato fries are a better option. Although they're still fried and have a lot of salt, they're also packed with beta carotene.
- If your restaurant meal is not all that healthy, keep things balanced with healthier foods, like more vegetables and fruit, at the next meal or snack.

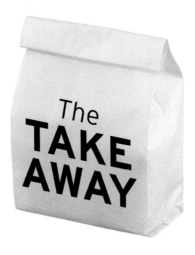

The **TAKE AWAY**

Ask how items are prepared. A side order of seasonal vegetables could be swimming in fat if the broccoli is sautéed in butter. You can always request that food be prepared without added fat—but it will be too late if it's already on the table.

Get all sauces and dressings on the side so you can control how they're drizzled on your meal. Many can add upwards of 100 calories; almost all will deliver a wallop of sodium.

Pack up half your meal to take home, even before you start digging in. Most restaurant portions are at least two times—and as many as eight times—bigger than recommended serving sizes.

Or ask for a half portion of your meal. Research has shown that people tend to eat as much as 40% more when they dine out. So eating half of a restaurant's portion size is probably the amount you would serve yourself at home.

Choose when to indulge if you dine out regularly. If a meal is an obligatory office lunch, then calories should count more than taste. If it's your birthday dinner, savour every bite.

AT
THE BAR

The bar. It's that hallowed place where men go to drink beer, to share a laugh and to indulge in some back-slapping boy time. Often, these trips revolve around sports. A UFC fight could be on the big-screen TVs, or a scrappy hockey match. Or maybe the bar is the place to meet up with the team after winning a baseball game.

Of course, nutrition will never be top of mind when the guys go out. But if slurping down pub grub is a weekly occurrence, then that barely-there six-pack is in danger of turning into a jiggly extra 6 pounds.

Bar food usually gets labelled as "starters." The term is misleading. It makes us think a basket of wings is a snack, something to nibble on before the real meal comes. In fact, most starters pack more of a calorific punch than an entree. That's the bad news. The good news is that by ordering off the main menu you can get an equally manly, equally indulgent meal *and* save calories. Calories that can go towards a pint of beer. Or preserving your physique.

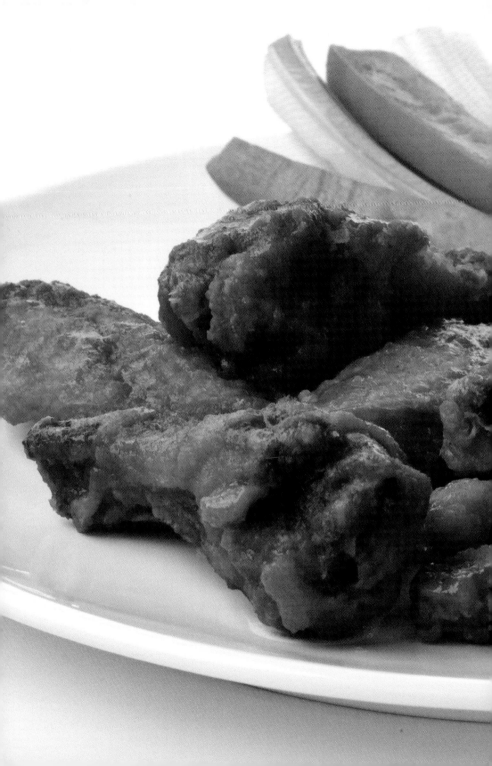

Kelsey's Classic Chicken Wings

For many men, a pound of wings and a pint of beer is the cornerstone of a night out. These crispy, juicy, salty nuggets of meat have many things going for them. They can be eaten without cutlery. They tap into caveman consciousness. They are as drool-inducing as bacon. Meat, not vegetables, is the main attraction.

DANGER ZONE: At Kelsey's, the Buffalo chicken sandwich with a side Caesar salad has 950 calories, 56 grams of fat and 1,650 mg of sodium.

SMART SWAP: If you *must* have wings at Kelsey's, beware the sauces. This is where the stratospheric levels of sodium lurk. Six of the nine offered sauces have more than 1,000 mg of sodium per serving—and four have more sodium than you need in a whole day. Asking your server to use half the usual amount of sauce can help. Or, if you can forgo the super salty hot sauce, ask for your wings to be coated in honey garlic sauce. It has a much more reasonable 360 mg of sodium.

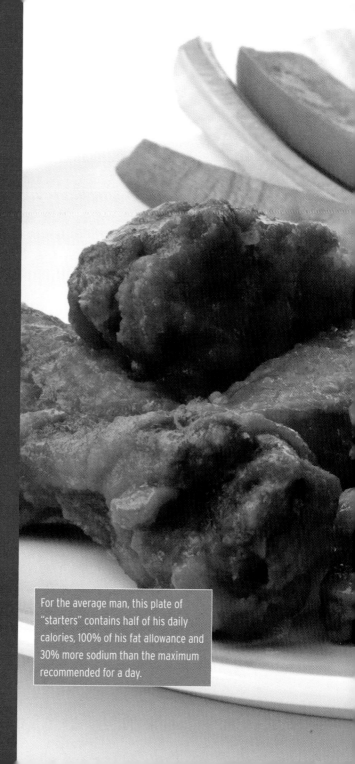

KELSEY'S CLASSIC CHICKEN WINGS

8 CHICKEN WINGS
Calories: 1,020
Fat: 68 grams
Carbohydrates: 3 grams
Protein: 97 grams
Sodium: 280 mg
Salt shakes: 7

HOT SAUCE
Calories: 80
Fat: 6 grams
Carbohydrates: 5 grams
Protein: 0.5 grams
Sodium: 2,330 mg
Salt shakes: 58

CELERY AND CARROT STICKS
Calories: 20
Fat: 0 grams
Carbohydrates: 5 grams
Protein: 1 gram
Sodium: 55 mg
Salt shakes: 1

BLUE CHEESE DRESSING
Calories: 150
Fat: 16 grams
Carbohydrates: 1 gram
Protein: 1 gram
Sodium: 300 mg
Salt shakes: 7 1/2

TOTAL
Calories: 1,270
Fat: 90 grams
Carbohydrates: 14 grams
Protein: 99.5 grams
Sodium: 2,965 mg
Salt shakes: 74

For the average man, this plate of "starters" contains half of his daily calories, 100% of his fat allowance and 30% more sodium than the maximum recommended for a day.

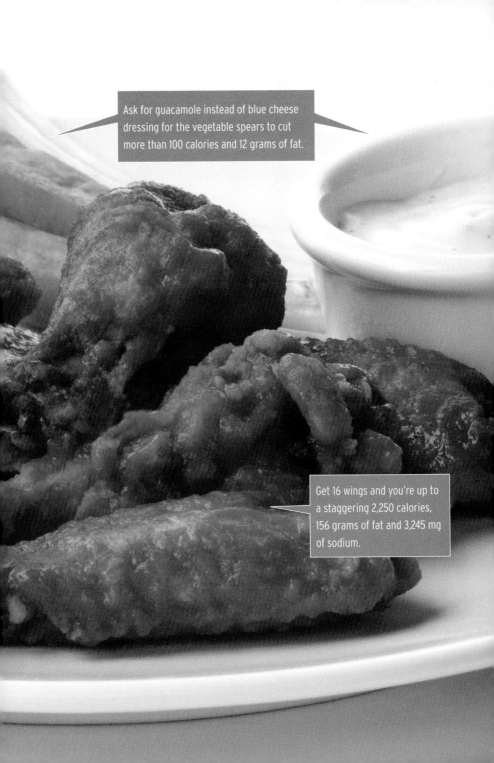

Boston Pizza Southwest potato skins

Barbeque sauce, crisp bacon, spicy chicken, two kinds of cheese. These are the ingredients that make a man's mouth water. They are also the things that turn a potato from a nutrient-rich vegetable that usually has fewer than 200 calories and minuscule amounts of fat and sodium into a greasy pile of calories.

A better choice is to split a pepperoni and mushroom pizza with your friend. Three pieces from a medium pizza has 600 calories, 21 grams of fat and 1,200 mg of sodium.

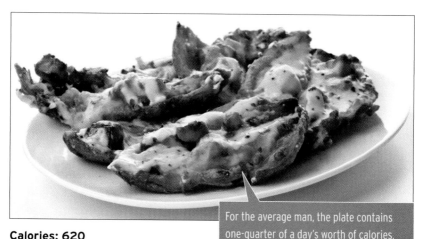

For the average man, the plate contains one-quarter of a day's worth of calories, one-third of a day's worth of fat and 85% of his maximum daily sodium allotment.

Calories: 620
Fat: 32 grams
Carbohydrates: 61 grams
Protein: 26 grams
Sodium: 2,010 mg
Salt shakes: 50

Jack Astor's grilled chicken quesadilla

You ate a burger for lunch, so you want something light at the bar. The grilled chicken quesadilla at Jack Astor's seems like the smart choice, with its grilled chicken, flour tortilla and tomato-heavy pico de gallo.

But this harmless-sounding starter clocks in with as many calories and almost as much fat as a 1/2 lb Double Baconator Burger from Wendy's. Though not healthy by any means, the quesadilla is still one of the lighter choices on Jack's calorie-heavy menu. Only the soups and some salads have fewer calories.

DANGER ZONE: Jack Astor's danger zone is more like a burning wasteland. Many, many things on this menu could be listed here. A pound of chicken wings with hot sauce has one and a half days' worth of fat. The chicken parmigiana contains 1,751 calories and as much fat as 12 cups of vanilla ice cream. The steak fajitas with redeye sauce has 6,402 mg of sodium—more than four times the sodium your body needs in a day!

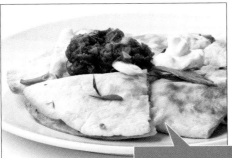

Calories: 946

Fat: 53 grams

Carbohydrates: 57 grams

Protein: 61 grams

Sodium: 1,831 mg

Salt shakes: 46

For the average man, the quesadilla has 40% of his daily calories, more than half of his fat intake and about three-quarters of the maximum sodium allotment.

MONTANA'S COOKHOUSE MUCHO NACHOS

These chili-smothered nachos will surely melt the heart of any meat-loving man. Along with spicy chili, baked beans, melted cheese, a "wackload" of diced tomato and green onion, and tiny bits of jalapeño grace the mound of nachos. Of course, the platter is served with sour cream and salsa.

No one would mistake this for health food. But would you guess that it has as much fat as 40 strips of bacon? And more calories than a large Bacon Double Cheeseburger pizza from Pizza Pizza? Your best bet here is to split the nachos—four ways. You're still eating the same amount of fat as in 10 strips of bacon and the calorie equivalent of one-quarter of a large meat-covered pizza. But divvying the nacho plate renders it a reasonable, rather than an outrageous, indulgence.

Calories: 2,450
Fat: 133 grams
Carbohydrates: 223 grams
Protein: 87 grams
Sodium: 3,500 mg
Salt shakes: 87 1/2

SMART SWAP: The Cookhouse Top Sirloin dinner. That's an 8-ounce top sirloin served with coleslaw, baked beans and fries for 920 calories, 40 grams of fat and 2,070 mg of sodium. This is a huge meal, but you could eat it twice over and still have consumed fewer calories and less fat than what's piled on the plate of nachos.

1 order of Montana's Cookhouse Mucho Nachos

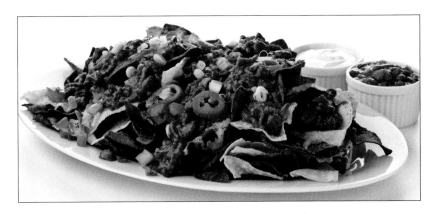

EQUALS

40 strips of bacon

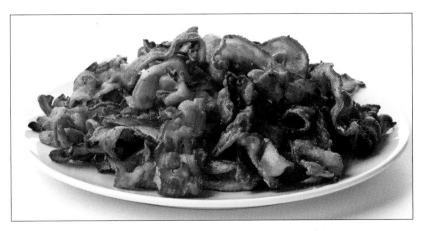

The nacho plate has as much fat as 40 strips of bacon.

Beer

Beer bellies are due to downing pints, of course. But the mindless snacking and wing eating that usually accompanies a trip to the bar also contributes to a growing girth.

The more you drink, the more likely you'll consume extra calories. Mostly because making wise food choices won't be top of mind when your mind is swimming from the suds.

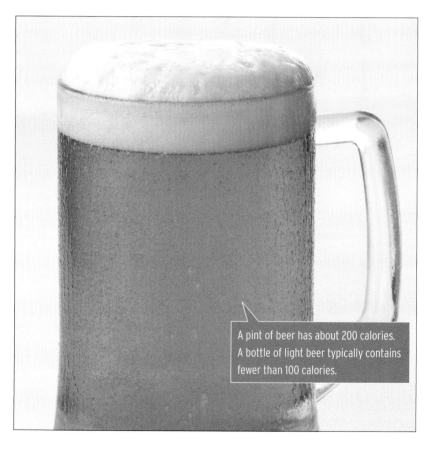

A pint of beer has about 200 calories. A bottle of light beer typically contains fewer than 100 calories.

Hooters Buffalo shrimp

Food isn't the first reason men sidle into a Hooters. They may say they go for the wings—just as men read *Playboy* for the articles—but it's the attributes of the servers, not the food next to their serviette, that holds their attention.

A popular "Hooterizer" is fried butterflied shrimp shaken in your favourite wing sauce. In a place where size matters, this appetizer is surprisingly small.

SMART SWAP: It's hard to say what would be better, since Hooters doesn't provide nutrition information. But getting shrimp that hasn't been dunked in a deep fryer can only improve the nutrition numbers. Just skip the butter sauce.

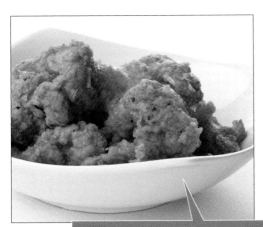

Calories: 347
Fat: 18 grams
Carbohydrates: 42 grams
Protein: 5 grams
Sodium: 1,406 mg
Salt shakes: 35

For the average man, this "Hooterizer" contains a minimal amount of his daily calories (18%) and the 18 grams of fat is just 20% of the recommended daily allotment. So not so bad—thanks to a true-sized appetizer. But the sodium—almost as much as your body needs in a day—sinks the shrimp.

Homemade nachos

At most restaurants, a platter of nachos will ring in with 2,000 calories, more than 100 grams of fat and two days' worth of sodium; nutrition numbers that humble even a Double Big Mac.

Not so with a platter of homemade nachos. With the right kind of tortilla chips and a smart selection of toppings, nachos assembled in your kitchen can have 75% fewer calories, 85% less fat and one-third less sodium.

27 Baked! Tostitos Scoops
   tortilla chips
50 grams grilled chicken
   breast, chopped
1/4 cup diced red pepper

1/4 cup shredded reduced-fat
   cheddar cheese
1 green onion, chopped
1/2 cup chunky salsa

Arrange tortilla chips on an oven-safe platter. Scatter chicken breast, red pepper and shredded cheese over top. Broil for 2 to 3 minutes, until cheese has melted. Top with green onion and serve with salsa.

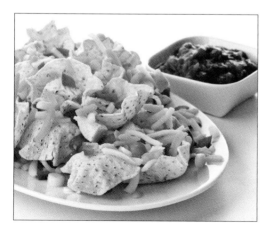

Calories: 460
Fat: 15 grams
Carbohydrates: 54 grams
Protein: 31 grams
Sodium: 1,498 mg
Salt shakes: 37

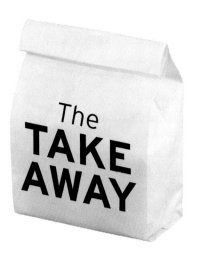

The
**TAKE
AWAY**

Consider starters the main attraction.
Most starters on bar menus pack 100 calories per big bite.

Split, split, split. And split some more.
Sharing the calories will help offset the dietary damage that can
be done while munching bar snacks and talking hockey.

Skim the full menu to see if something else
sparks your fancy. Often, entrees will offer more substance
and more nutrition for fewer calories.

Skip the drive-thru. Clearly, your favourite bar food
is an indulgence, so think about skipping other treats the rest
of the day. And maybe the day after, too.

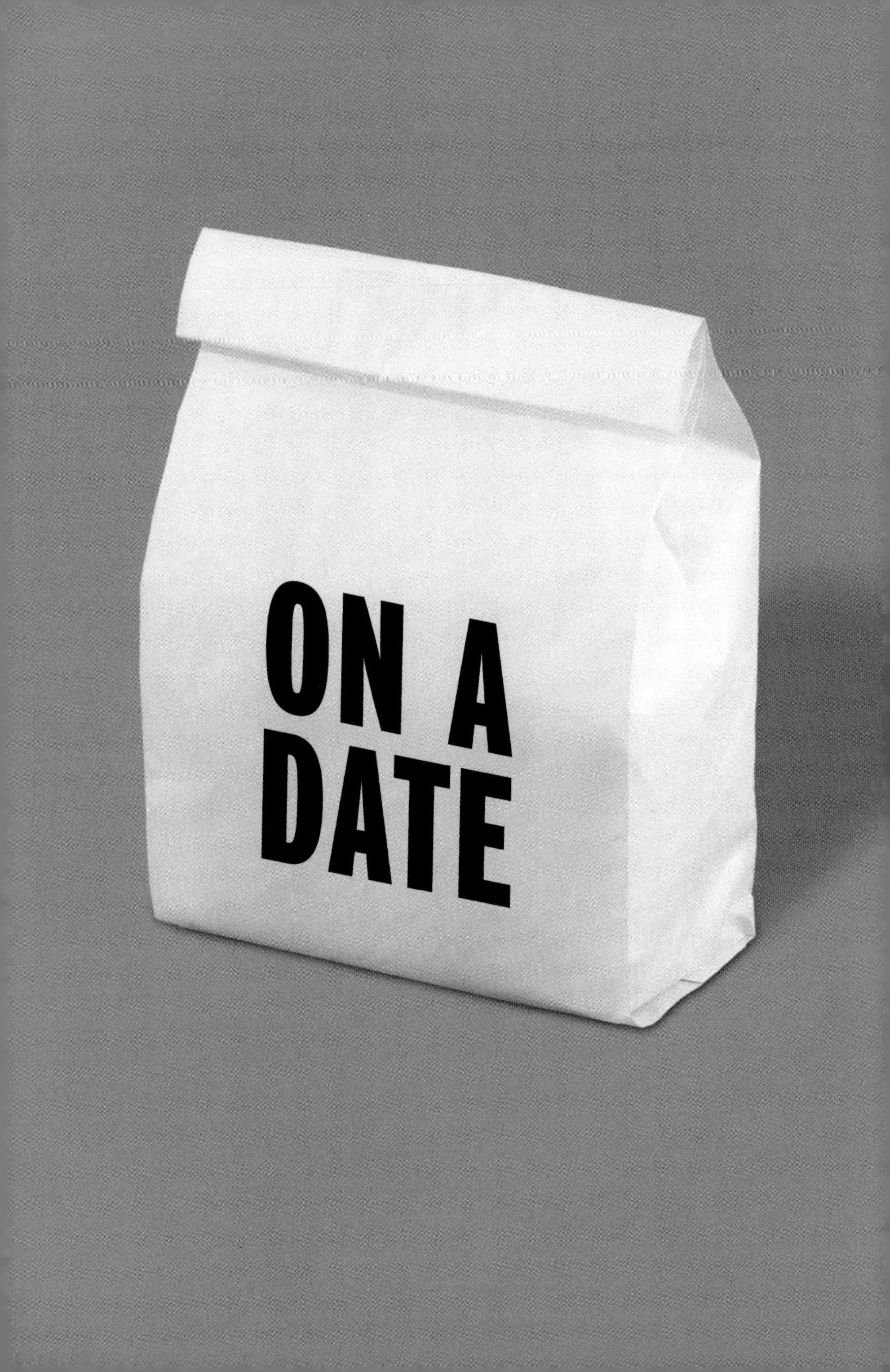
ON A
DATE

Whether it's your first date or your 101st time out as an established couple, you'll likely end up sitting down and sharing a treat. It may be a luscious dessert at a fancy restaurant to mark a relationship milestone. Or a quick bite at the mall before embarking on a joint shopping expedition. Or a snack in a cozy coffee house after a chilly stroll in the park.

Since a date should be decidedly stress-free, you shouldn't worry too much about calories (even though many of the date-worthy foods featured here are riddled with them). That's why splitting makes so much sense. Plus there are lots of fun ways you and your date can burn off those pesky calories. Besides, you know, the obvious.

\>

Cineplex Entertainment medium bag of popcorn with butter topping

Like Rhett Butler and Scarlett O'Hara, movies and popcorn are an iconic pairing. It's hard to have one without the other. Especially when taking in a flick at the local movie theatre, where the seductive scent of buttery popcorn lingers over the concession stand. It's nearly impossible to resist that bag of kernels. Too bad the secret ingredient is fat—and several dashes of salt.

In 2007, Cineplex Entertainment switched to a proprietary popping oil called Vegetol, which includes canola oil and artificial butter flavour. The new oil is lower in calories, fat, saturated fat and trans fat than traditional coconut oil, but this medium bag from Cineplex still holds about a day's worth of fat.* For some of you, that fact will be as frightening as a 3-D horror film. Others might just say, "Frankly, my dear, I don't give a damn."

Calories: 1,212

Fat: 81 grams

Carbohydrates: 105 grams

Protein: 16 grams

Sodium: 744 mg

Salt shakes: 19

SMART SWAP: If every Friday night is date night at the movies, consider skipping the butter topping. That will save about 300 calories and 50 grams of fat. Or, walk right past the concession stand. Without that bag of popcorn, you and your date can sit that much closer.

---

*As tested by an independent lab. Cineplex data, which may differ, is not readily accessible.

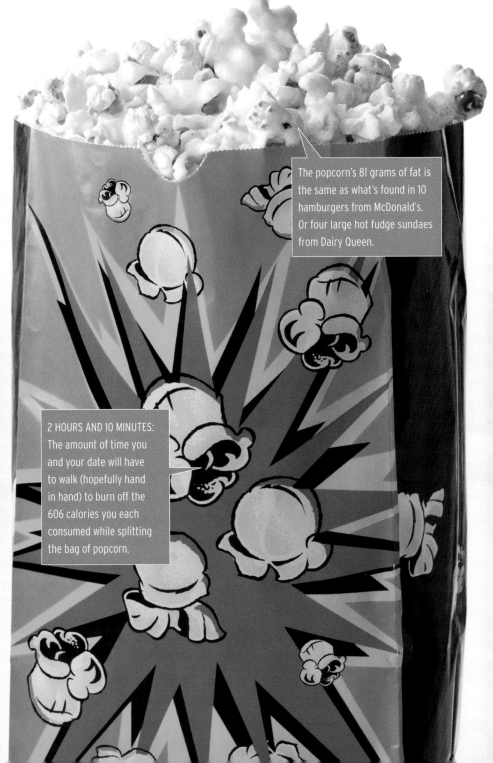

Cineplex Entertainment nacho tray with salsa dip and cheese dip

It's like the wizards of animation responsible for the latest blockbuster cartoon have created the nachos served at theatre concession stands. Each chip is perfectly round. They often come beautifully arranged in a handy black tray. The cheese sauce is an impossibly bright electric orange.

The calories, too, are a little unreal. Even if you split it with your squeeze, the nacho tray contains the number of calories you should aim for in a meal.*

Calories: 1,002
Fat: 46 grams
Carbohydrates: 134 grams
Protein: 13 grams
Sodium: 1,748 mg
Salt shakes: 44

DANGER ZONE: In some worlds, a medium pop is, well, a medium-sized drink. At Cineplex, the medium soda contains 1 litre of pop. If you choose Coca-Cola, a medium drink will cost you 450 calories and 118 grams of sugar. That's like crunching on 28 sugar cubes. Knowing that, why not pick up a bottle of water to quench your thirst?

*As tested by an independent lab. Cineplex data, which may differ, is not readily accessible.

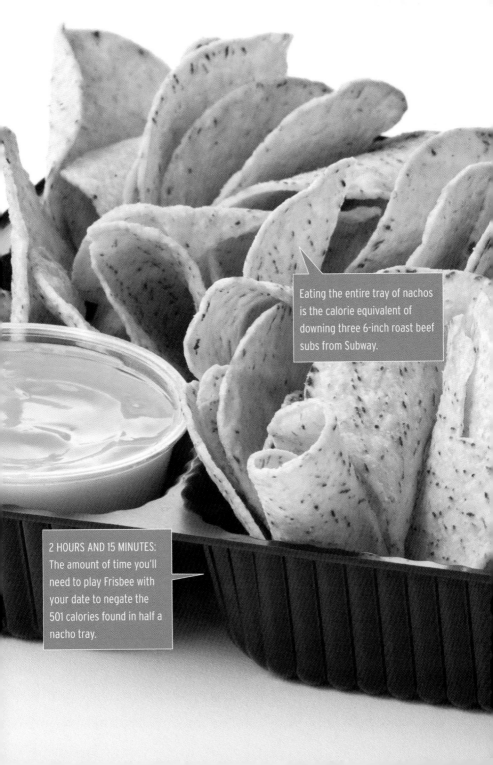

Eating the entire tray of nachos is the calorie equivalent of downing three 6-inch roast beef subs from Subway.

2 HOURS AND 15 MINUTES: The amount of time you'll need to play Frisbee with your date to negate the 501 calories found in half a nacho tray.

Rocky Mountain Chocolate Factory Skor-covered caramel apple

The caramel apples dreamed up by the folks at Rocky Mountain are much more than Granny Smiths dunked in caramelized sugar. These ones come rolled in pieces of candy bar, covered in snowy white marshmallow and swathed in layers of chocolate—along with the requisite coating of caramel.

While choosing from the impressive crop of flavours, including rocky road, s'more and cheesecake, you and your date may be tempted to get one each. It's an *apple*—how bad can it be? Unfortunately, by the time it has rolled down the Rocky Mountain, a Skor-covered caramel apple has more in common with candy than fruit.

Calories: 734
Fat: 33 grams
Carbohydrates: 102 grams
Protein: 8 grams
Sodium: 280 mg
Salt shakes: 7

SMART SWAP: If you and your date have wandered into the Rocky Mountain Chocolate Factory for a sweet treat, consider bypassing the caramel apples for the chocolate-coated caramels. Savouring a selection of two or three will likely do less calorie damage.

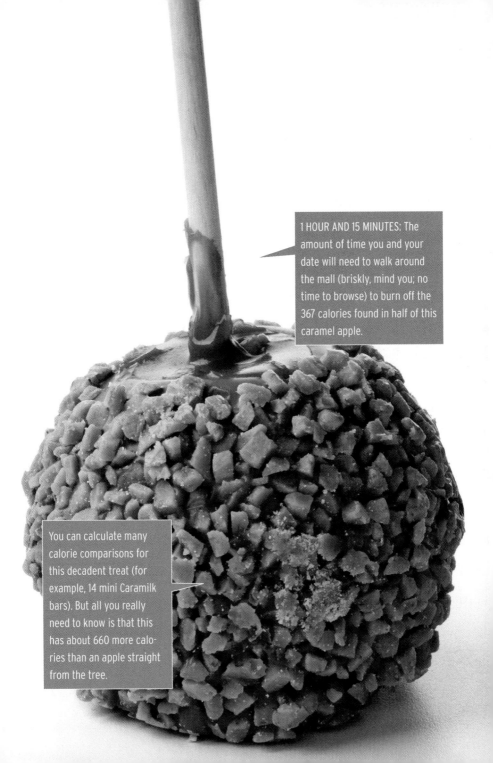

1 HOUR AND 15 MINUTES: The amount of time you and your date will need to walk around the mall (briskly, mind you; no time to browse) to burn off the 367 calories found in half of this caramel apple.

You can calculate many calorie comparisons for this decadent treat (for example, 14 mini Caramilk bars). But all you really need to know is that this has about 660 more calories than an apple straight from the tree.

Earls Kitchen & Bar
New York–style cheesecake

Most of us know a dish made with cream cheese won't be considered health food. But who would guess that this modest slice of cheesecake, topped with blueberry compote, would clock in at 730 calories and nearly 50 grams of fat? That's like finishing your meal with . . . another whole meal. This dessert definitely requires two forks.

Calories: 730
Fat: 49 grams
Carbohydrates: 59
Protein: 13 grams
Sodium: 530 mg
Salt shakes: 13

MEGAN'S TIP: It doesn't take a nutrition genius to know desserts are stuffed with calories. But I had no idea, until I started scouring nutrition numbers, the ones served at restaurants typically have at least 500 calories. And many are more likely to contain 700 or 800. For me, that's way too much calorie investment for a sweet. I have always split dessert when dining out—mostly because I'm already stuffed. My new dining-out strategy is to splurge on dessert only if the restaurant has its own pastry chef or is known for its after-dinner treats. I don't mind devoting a few hundred calories to something truly delectable. And I still ask for two forks.

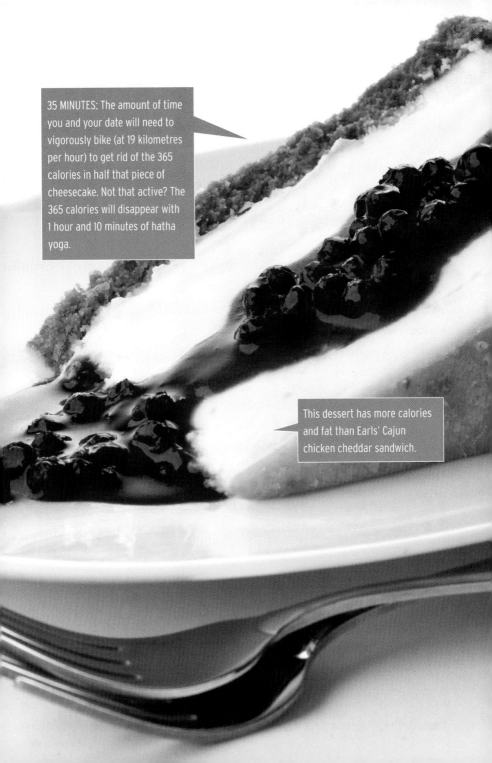

35 MINUTES: The amount of time you and your date will need to vigorously bike (at 19 kilometres per hour) to get rid of the 365 calories in half that piece of cheesecake. Not that active? The 365 calories will disappear with 1 hour and 10 minutes of hatha yoga.

This dessert has more calories and fat than Earls' Cajun chicken cheddar sandwich.

CINNABON CARAMEL PECANBON

Cinnabon's world-famous cinnamon rolls smell as good as they taste. Their aroma is so intoxicating that people buy Cinnabon-spiked candles to give their home that sweet, straight-from-the-oven, cinnamon scent.

If you can be content with just smelling Cinnabon rolls, resist taking a bite. A Cinnabon—especially the caramel pecan version—is also a calorie bomb. Splitting it will help diffuse some of the danger.

CINNABON CARAMEL PECANBON

Calories: 1,080
Fat: 50 grams
Carbohydrates: 147 grams (including 76 grams sugars)
Protein: 14 grams
Sodium: 960 mg
Salt shakes: 24

SMART SWAPS: This treat can be redeemed. A Minibon Roll has 350 calories and 14 grams of fat—two-thirds fewer calories and grams of fat than the Caramel Pecanbon. Even better, order a pack of four Caramel Pecanbon Bites to split with your date. That way you satisfy your sweet tooth and consume just 276 calories and 13.5 grams of fat.

1 Cinnabon Caramel Pecanbon

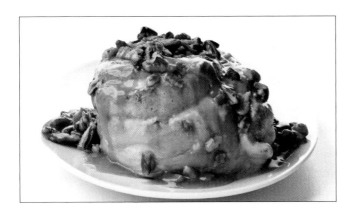

EQUALS

1/3 of a cup of sugar and 1/2 a stick of butter

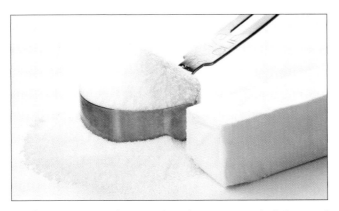

A single Caramel Pecanbon has as much fat as a half stick of butter and the equivalent of a heaping 1/3 cup sugar.

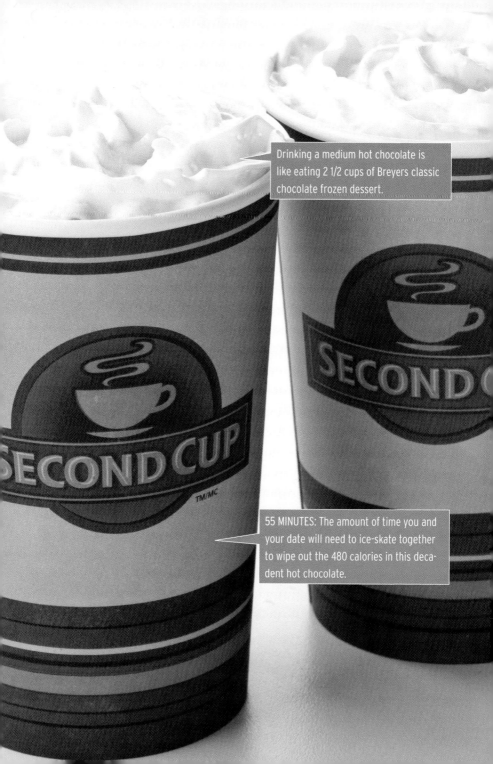

Second Cup hot chocolate

After ice-skating with your sweetie, you may be tempted to warm up with a creamy hot chocolate—it tastes like dessert in a cup. Especially with whipped cream floating on top. Calorie-wise, it resembles dessert, too. And a single 16-ounce hot chocolate from Second Cup packs a surprising 22 grams of fat.

16-OUNCE (500 ML) HOT CHOCOLATE MADE
WITH 2% MILK AND TOPPED WITH WHIPPED CREAM

Calories: 480
Fat: 22 grams
Carbohydrates: 60 grams (including 50 grams sugars)
Protein: 13 grams
Sodium: 450 mg
Salt shakes: 11

SMART SWAP: It's a little awkward to split a mug of hot chocolate. So instead of sharing this treat, why not downsize? Second Cup offers an 8-ounce (250 mL) hot chocolate. This wee-sized indulgence is equally romantic on a wintery night. With skim milk and whipped cream (can't get rid of all the luxuries), it saves you almost 200 calories and 8 grams of fat.

Decadent—but not deadly—delicacies for your date

At the mall

Instead of a fruit dipped in caramel, look for a fruit- and caramel-filled crepe. At Crepe Delicious, the Caramel Apple crepe—made with sliced apples and caramel and topped with walnuts—has 269 calories and 5 grams of fat. Split this for a tasty—and healthy—treat.

At the movies

Instead of munching on popcorn, choose a box of Junior Mints to split with your date. A few handfuls of the candy will net you only 170 calories and 3 grams of fat.

At the coffee shop

Instead of a hot chocolate, sip a non-fat latte. A medium-sized latte made with skim milk at Second Cup has 140 calories and 1 gram of fat. With chocolate sprinkles scattered on top, this drink can still feel sinful.

At the fancy restaurant

Instead of an 800 calorie slice of cake, order a piece of biscotti and a cup of decaf coffee or herbal tea. You will get the satisfaction of a sweet without giving up half of your day's worth of calories. A plate of seasonal fruit will also round out a meal nicely. And a single scoop of ice cream will satisfy a sweet tooth without breaking the calorie bank.

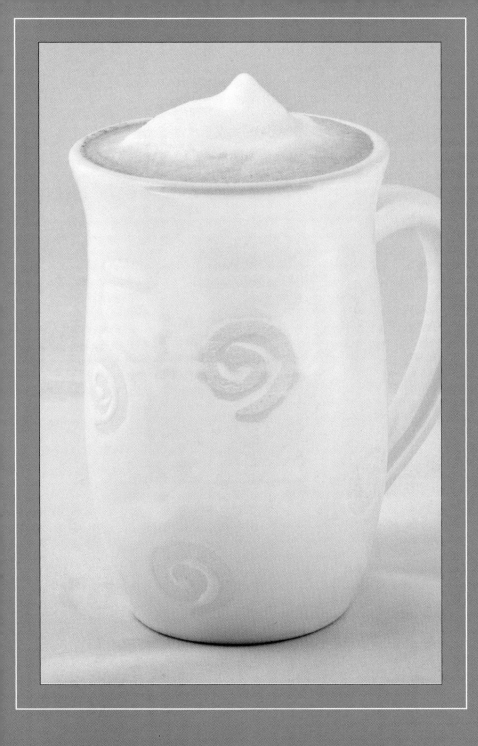

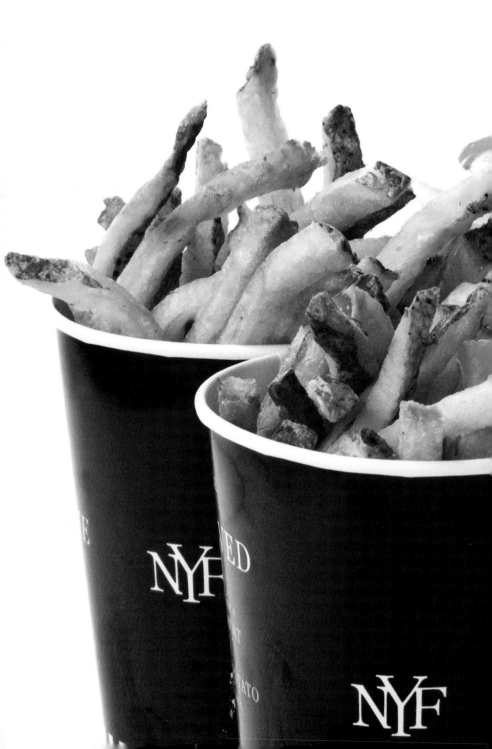

New York Fries

French fries wouldn't usually be considered traditional date food. But New York Fries, which hails from Canada, not the Big Apple, markets a french fry meal for two. You each get a regular order of fries and a drink. Then you get to split the cheese sauce and the gravy. Dunking together, very sweet.

Even if you treat this spread of fries as a meal, the 872 calories is more than what you should be eating in a single sitting.

SMART SWAP: Rather than just sharing the sauce, what if you split a regular fries, order two bottles of water and continue to double dip in the gravy? Going splits this way means your trip to New York Fries costs only a reasonable 312 calories and 13.5 grams of fat. Plus, you'll consume a lot less sodium.

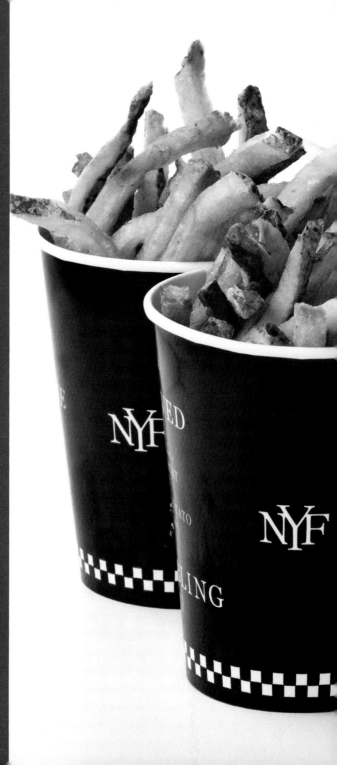

NEW YORK FRIES

FRENCH FRIES,
REGULAR SIZE
Calories: 580
Fat: 27 grams
Carbohydrates: 70 grams
Protein: 7 grams
Sodium: 125 mg
Salt shakes: 3

CHEESE SAUCE,
REGULAR SIZE
Calories: 100
Fat: 1.5 grams
Carbohydrates: 19 grams
Protein: 1 gram
Sodium: 780 mg
Salt shakes: 19 1/2

GRAVY, REGULAR SIZE
Calories: 45
Fat: 0.5 grams
Carbohydrates: 9 grams
Protein: 1 gram
Sodium: 562 mg
Salt shakes: 14

PEPSI,
REGULAR SIZE (500 ML)
Calories: 220
Carbohydrates: 29 grams
(all sugars)

TOTAL PER PERSON
Calories: 872
Fat: 28 grams
Carbohydrates: 119 grams
Protein: 8 grams
Sodium: 796 mg
Salt shakes: 20

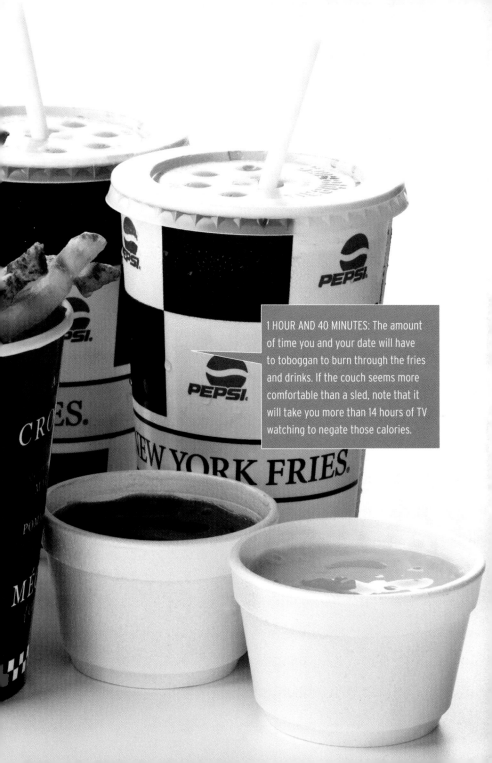

1 HOUR AND 40 MINUTES: The amount of time you and your date will have to toboggan to burn through the fries and drinks. If the couch seems more comfortable than a sled, note that it will take you more than 14 hours of TV watching to negate those calories.

Let's stay in

Why go out when you can curl up on the couch, snuggled close to your date? Staying at home with your squeeze has many benefits. You can set the mood with candles and music. You can watch a classic movie that will get heart-strings strumming. You'll be able to chat without having to yell over a crowd of chattering strangers. And treats cooked up in your kitchen won't settle so firmly around your waist. Here are some ideas for date-worthy nibbles:

Make a big bowl of homemade popcorn: 2 cups of air-popped popcorn has just 66 calories and only 1 gram of fat and 1 gram of sodium. Shake with a tablespoon or so of freshly grated Parmesan cheese, or toss with a dash of cinnamon and sugar. The same amount of microwave popcorn with butter flavour has about 150 calories, 9 grams of fat and 230 mg of sodium.

What's more romantic than strawberries dipped in melted chocolate? A cup of strawberries dipped in 1/3 cup melted chocolate has about 170 calories.

Sip on gourmet coffee made by adding a glug of Irish whiskey or a sweet liqueur to your mug.

Share a banana split made with more fruit than ice cream.

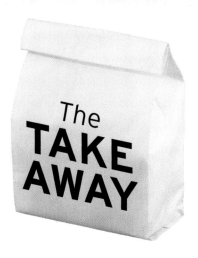

The
**TAKE
AWAY**

Sharing is good with a date. You each get all the taste of a treat for half the calories. In addition to divvying up calories, sharing a meal or treat with a friend may boost your happiness. Research has shown that people who share release oxytocin, a hormone that influences happiness and is known to relieve stress and boost immune function.

Dining with another person—especially one whom you want to get to know better—means you may be more focused on chatting than eating. By slowing down your eating, you're more likely to take in fewer calories.

Sharing is good with yourself. If you are craving a treat, consider enjoying half (or a third) and putting the remainder in the fridge for the following day.

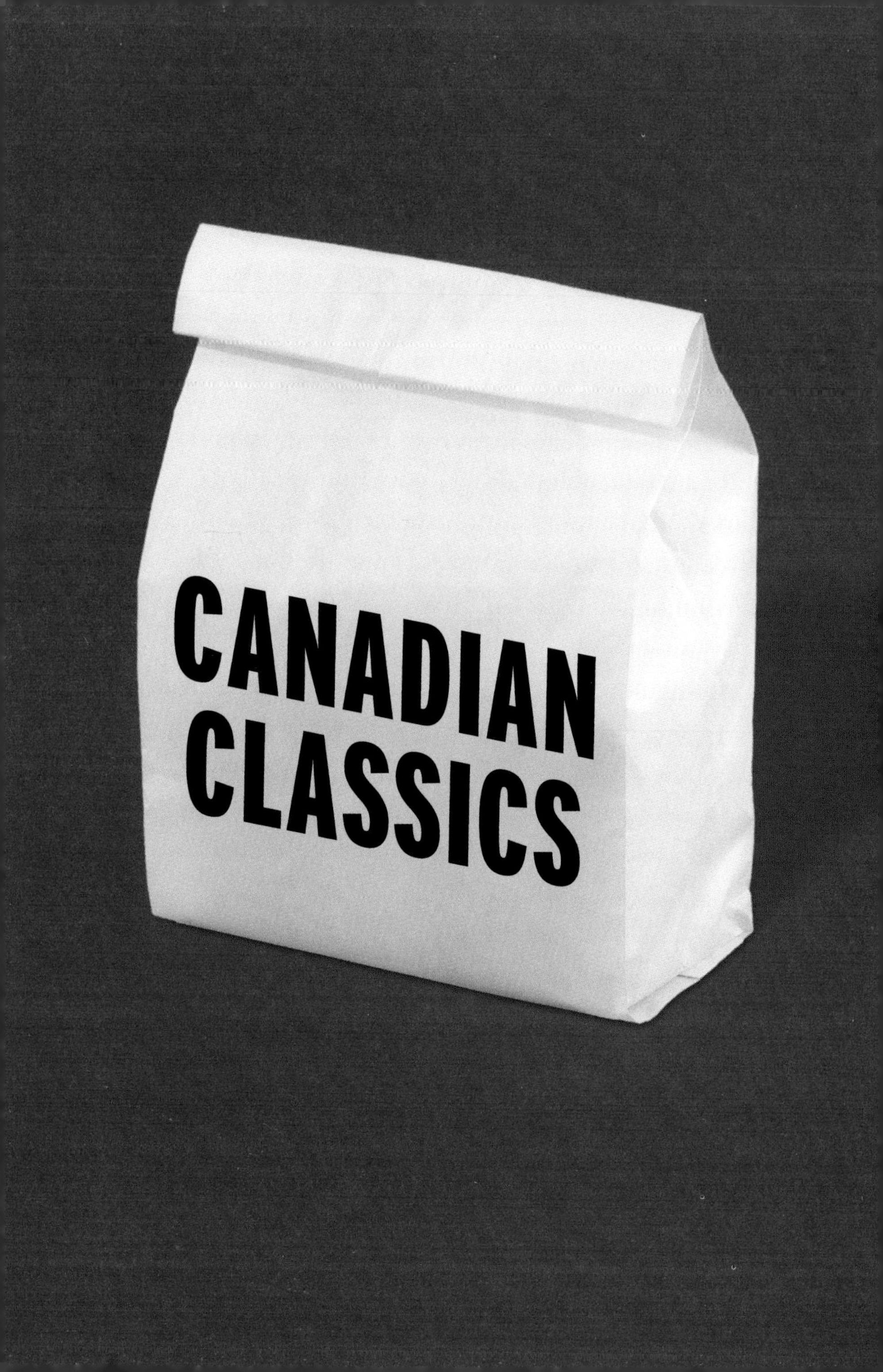
CANADIAN
CLASSICS

There are many things that make Canada our home and native land. Oceans and mountains, lakes and prairies, sweeping tundra and swaths of harder-than-steel Canadian Shield bedrock. Hockey played on ponds and rinks and roads. Toques. Tim Hortons. Publicly funded health care. The CBC.

There is also our indomitable spirit and quiet pride. Our welcoming borders. Our winters. Our tight-knit communities and world-class cities. And, of course, our food. While some may argue Canada does not have a single national dish, there are dozens of foods unique to this country. Each of us has a favourite. In this chapter you will get a nutritional peek at some iconic Canadian foods. It's not an exhaustive list—not by a long shot. Nor is it an attempt to steer you away from the decadent dishes. Think of this last chapter as a fun and friendly FYI.

After all, much-loved foods should be savoured. This is why there are no proposed tweaks to cut fat or suggested swaps to whittle calories. (Would poutine be poutine without the gravy?) And since many of the following foods can't be eaten in quick succession—unless you have access to a private jet—they are clearly once-in-a-while treats. So enjoy some of the best things Canada has to offer. Just don't go for seconds.

Butter tart, Dee's General Store, Valens, Ontario

The small community of Valens, Ontario, may be the butter tart capital of Canada—thanks to a small general store there.

It's hard to be precise about these things. But Dee's General Store has sold more than 1.4 million butter tarts since the first batch was baked in 1986. All of them were handmade by Dee and her small contingent of loyal bakers in the back of her gas station's general store.

What makes these butter tarts better than others? Dee claims it's their size; she makes them in muffin tins, not tart pans, so they are especially hefty. To further entice butter tart fanatics, she also offers more than a dozen flavours, from caramel to coconut, from café mocha to candy bar. And it might also have something to do with their over-the-top tag line: Dee refers to them as "butter tarts to die for."

While no one has keeled over from eating a tart, people have driven more than six hours to have a taste.

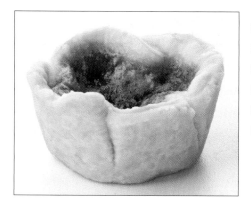

Calories: 340
Fat: 20 grams
Carbohydrates: 36 grams
Protein: 3 grams
Sodium: 141 mg
Salt shakes: 3 1/2

BeaverTail, Byward Market, Ottawa, Ontario

It is a frostily cold afternoon and you are skating along Ottawa's frozen Rideau Canal hand in hand with your sweetheart. What could be a better, more welcome treat than a cup of hot chocolate and a warm BeaverTail?

For those who don't know, this Canadian creation is made with sweet, whole-wheat dough that has been hand-stretched to resemble a beaver's tail and then popped into vat of bubbling oil.

The first was sold at Ottawa's Byward Market. Now you can find BeaverTails across Canada, including in Banff and Halifax, Collingwood and Cavendish, Montreal, Moncton and Mont-Tremblant. In winter, when the Rideau Canal becomes a giant skating rink, BeaverTails are sold from small red huts along the edge of the frozen waterway.

It's hard to know whether they taste best topped with cinnamon and sugar or with chocolate hazelnut sauce or maple butter. You could try one of each to find out.

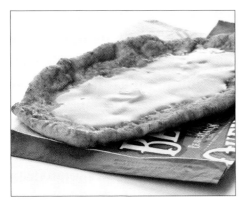

BEAVERTAIL TOPPED WITH MAPLE BUTTER
Calories: 333
Fat: 9 grams
Carbohydrates: 58 grams
Protein: 5 grams
Sodium: 346 mg
Salt shakes: 9

McLobster, McDonald's, Maritimes

Yes, the rumours are true: there is a McLobster season at McDonald's. But only in Atlantic Canada, only at certain locations and only at certain times of the year.

A McLobster sounds a little like a monster from a children's horror film. But the strange-sounding sandwich isn't scary. It's a simple creation. Just a creamy mixture of pink lobster pieces and chopped celery stuffed into a fluffy white bun.

That McDonald's offers up a fast-food take on a traditional lobster roll will undoubtedly make some people chuckle. But the sandwich has a contingent of devout fans who dash to their local Mickey D's when the McLobster comes to town.

Calories: 205
Fat: 3 grams
Carbohydrates: 24 grams
Protein: 20 grams
Sodium: 667 mg
Salt shakes: 17

Donair, King of Donair, Halifax, Nova Scotia

A small family-owned eatery on Halifax's Quinpool Road was the first in Canada to serve a donair. That was in 1973. Since then, thousands have devoured the Mediterranean-style pita made with spiced beef, chopped onion, diced tomato and sweet, sugar-spiked garlic sauce.

Donairs are now found in sandwich shops and pizza parlours across Canada. But the King of Donair claims its world-famous sandwich can never be duplicated. Its legions of admirers agree.

Calories: 592
Fat: 31 grams
Carbohydrates: 56 grams
Protein: 22 grams
Sodium: 1,142 mg
Salt shakes: 28 1/2

Chips, dressing and gravy, Rod's Restaurant, Clarenville, Newfoundland

Those of us who don't hail from the Rock are likely unfamiliar with chips, dressing and gravy. This Newfoundland specialty may sound like a version of poutine, that other oh-so-Canadian dish. But Newfoundlanders are swift to point out that their delicacy—served at almost every chip truck, gas station and mom-and-pop diner across the province—is distinctly different.

The perfect CDG is made with crisply fried chips—preferably homemade—topped with savoury dressing (or stuffing, to non-Atlantic Canadians) and smothered with thick, homestyle chicken gravy.

Although you can get CDG at some fry stands in other provinces, many Newfoundlanders maintain that chips, dressing and gravy tastes best when eaten in their hometowns in the company of friends.

Calories: 1,121
Fat: 51 grams
Carbohydrates: 144 grams
Protein: 21 grams
Sodium: 1,340 mg
Salt shakes: 33 1/2

Poutine, Chez Ashton, Quebec City, Quebec

Remember the first time you tried to explain poutine to an American friend? The description of french fries topped with cheese curds and gravy probably raised eyebrows or prompted a drawn-out *eeeewww*.

Sure, this Quebec specialty sounds strange to the uninitiated. But as anyone who has ever dug into a pile of poutine will attest, the ooey-gooey concoction is only strange in its addictiveness.

Chez Ashton in Quebec City claims to be the first to combine poutine's three key ingredients. The now-famous dish is served across Canada. But since many claim the original is best, here are nutrition numbers for the classic Canadian poutine.

Calories: 1,104
Fat: 58 grams
Carbohydrates: 113 grams
Protein: 32 grams
Sodium: 1,769 mg
Salt shakes: 44

Smoked meat sandwich, Schwartz's, Montreal, Quebec

If you are a visitor to Montreal and ask a local where to go for a smoked meat sandwich, chances are you will be directed to Schwartz's. The landmark restaurant, located on Montreal's historic Boulevard Saint-Laurent, claims to be the oldest delicatessen in Canada. Its loyal clientele includes rock stars, Hollywood celebrities and heads of state.

Take one bite of the towering sandwich stuffed with delicately thin slices of smoked meat and you will know why Schwartz's has been doing brisk business since 1928.

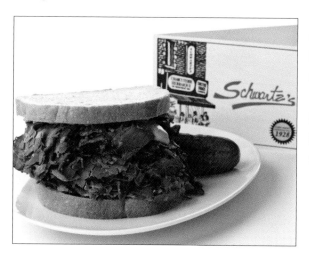

Calories: 410
Fat: 9 grams
Carbohydrates:
    23 grams
Protein: 60 grams
Sodium: 2,076 mg
Salt shakes: 52

Back bacon on a bun, Carousel Bakery, Toronto, Ontario

For more than 30 years, hungry market-goers have been lining up for Carousel Bakery's "world-famous" bacon on a bun. This unpretentious sandwich generates a slavish devotion in its admirers, who regularly flock to Toronto's vibrant St. Lawrence Market to get their bacon fix.

Almost every food magazine, travel rag and big city newspaper has raved about Carousel's bacon on a bun. It all becomes clear once you have had your first taste of the fried-to-perfection peameal bacon layered carefully in a warm, fresh-baked bun. Yum.

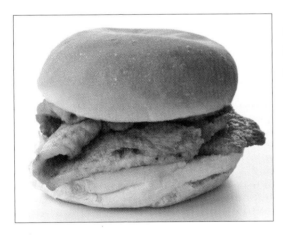

Calories: 494
Fat: 11 grams
Carbohydrates:
   52 grams
Protein: 46 grams
Sodium: 2,470 mg
Salt shakes: 62

Hot dog, Bay Street hot dog cart, Toronto, Ontario

Whether you are a tourist to Toronto or one of Bay Street's bustling bankers, it can be hard to resist the siren call of grilling street meat. And since there are more than 300 hot dog vendors in downtown Toronto, it's never a far walk to find a frank.

Menus don't differ. It's just hot dogs, sausages and veggie wieners on toasted egg buns. But vendors try to lure customers to their carts with sumptuous selections of garnishes and toppings. Yes, there is mustard, ketchup and relish. And you will find pickles, sauerkraut, chopped onion and diced tomato. But if you are lucky, you could stumble upon a cart that offers sliced olives—green and black—bacon bits, horseradish, pickled peppers and maybe even salty pieces of crumbled potato chips.

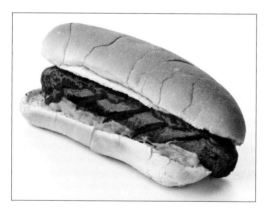

ALL-BEEF HOT DOG
WITH MUSTARD AND
KETCHUP AND BUN
Calories: 450
Fat: 21 grams
Carbohydrates: 47 grams
Protein: 18 grams
Sodium: 1,207 mg
Salt shakes: 30

Nip, Salisbury House, Winnipeg, Manitoba

You can get burgers in Winnipeg. You can also get nips. These famed sandwiches are sold at Salisbury House, a Winnipeg institution with 17 locations scattered across the city.

Sals, as it's commonly known, opened in 1931. The red-roofed restaurant was the first in the city to serve hamburgers, which owner Ralph Erwin decided to call "nips" because they were a smaller version of the Salisbury steak. They were an instant hit.

Since then, generations of Winnipeggers have eaten at Sals. And nips—ground beef patties served on homemade buns with "lots" of grilled onions—are still one of the most popular items on the menu.

So it's no surprise when Sals claims, "We put the NIP in Win-NIP-peg!"

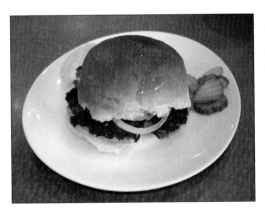

Calories: 377

Fat: 15 grams

Carbohydrates: 37 grams

Protein: 24 grams

Sodium: 331 mg

Salt shakes: 8

Photograph courtesy Terry Toews

Saskatoon berry pie, Saskatchewan

For those who grew up on the windswept prairies, a fresh-from-the-oven saskatoon berry pie is a beloved taste of home.

Some may argue that the piquant, deep purple berries taste best when eaten straight from a bush on a hot summer's day. Others emphatically claim the fruit is at its most sublime when stirred with sugar and baked into a pie.

Although saskatoon berry orchards are starting to spring up in eastern stretches of the country, it's not always easy to find the sharply sweet berries. That's why the farmers of Riverbend Plantation started shipping saskatoon berry pie filling from their Saskatoon-area orchard. Now any Canadian can get a taste of saskatoons, the queen berry of the prairies.

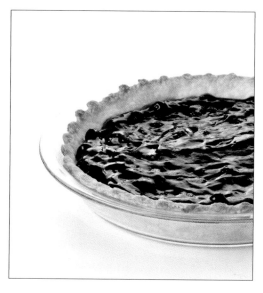

SASKATOON BERRY PIE made with a Compliments-brand frozen pie crust and 2 1/2 cups Riverbend Plantation saskatoon berry pie filling

Per 1/8 of pie

Calories: 228

Fat: 5 grams

Carbohydrates: 45 grams

Protein: 2 grams

Sodium: 70 mg

Salt shakes: 2

Perogies, Uncle Ed's Ukrainian Restaurant, Edmonton, Alberta

Sometimes all you crave is comfort food. In Edmonton, more times than not, the consoling dish will involve perogies.

The soul-satisfying dumplings can be found in many corners of the city. But Uncle Ed's Ukrainian Restaurant—at times called the "perogy palace"—is a mainstay for people craving pillowy perogies.

The homey, sit-down establishment offers all sorts of perogies. You can get them filled with onion or sauerkraut, stuffed with cottage or cheddar cheese and boiled, deep-fried or cooked crisp in a fry pan. All are served with—of course—sour cream, onions and homemade bacon bits.

Bud'mo! (That's how you'd say cheers in Ukrainian.)

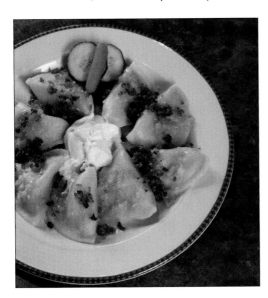

8 POTATO AND CHEDDAR CHEESE PEROGIES with sour cream, onions and bacon bits

Calories: 702
Fat: 24 grams
Carbohydrates: 102 grams
Protein: 19 grams
Sodium: 1,677 mg
Salt shakes: 42

Photograph courtesy Alexis Alchorn

Asado siopao (steamed pork bun), New Town Bakery, Vancouver, British Columbia

New Town Bakery has been selling Chinese and Filipino baked goods for more than 30 years. The family-run mini-chain has three locations: in Richmond, Surrey and Vancouver. But it's the clamorous bakery in Vancouver's Chinatown that reaps most of the attention.

Many claim New Town on Pender Street sells the best steamed buns on the west coast. Its *asado siopao*, or steamed pork buns, are among the most popular. The brilliantly white buns filled with sauce-covered slivers of barbequed pork are no two-bite snacks. They are liberal in size and generous in flavour. You get a lot of food for less than a toonie.

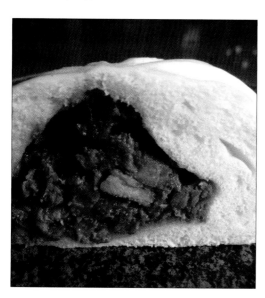

Per bun
Calories: 446
Fat: 14 grams
Carbohydrates: 64 grams
Protein: 14 grams
Sodium: 336 mg
Salt shakes: 8 1/2

Photograph courtesy Michael Seto

Official Nanaimo bar of Nanaimo, British Columbia

The Nanaimo bar originated in Nanaimo, British Columbia. There is no doubt about that. But according to the City of Nanaimo—and the folks there should know—no one knows *who* created this famous three-layered sweet. All we have is conjecture and speculation and many myths about the confection's mysterious origins.

To help settle the confusion, the mayor of Nanaimo in 1986 held a contest for the best Nanaimo bar recipe. There were more than 100 entrants. Joyce Hardcastle won. Her version of the West Coast concoction is seriously sweet. Give it a try. The recipe's on the next page.

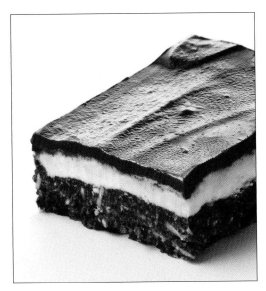

Per square
  (1/24th of recipe)
Calories: 205
Fat: 13 grams
Carbohydrates: 21 grams
Protein: 2 grams
Sodium: 54 mg
Salt shakes: 1

The official Nanaimo bar recipe

First Layer

1/2 cup unsalted butter

1/4 cup sugar

5 tablespoons cocoa powder

1 egg, beaten

1 1/4 cups graham wafer crumbs

1/2 cup finely chopped almonds

1 cup unsweetened shredded or flaked coconut

Melt the butter in the top of a double boiler, along with the sugar and cocoa. Add the egg, stirring to cook and thicken. Remove mixture from heat. Stir in the graham wafer crumbs, almonds and coconut. Press firmly into an ungreased 8- × 8-inch pan.

Second Layer

1/2 cup unsalted butter

2 tablespoons plus 2 teaspoons cream

2 tablespoons vanilla custard powder

2 cups icing sugar

Cream the butter with the cream, custard powder and icing sugar, until well mixed. Beat until light. Spread over bottom layer in pan.

4 1-ounce squares semi-sweet chocolate

2 tablespoons unsalted butter

Melt the chocolate and butter over low heat or in the top of a double boiler. Remove from heat and let cool. Once cool but still liquid, pour over second layer. Chill in refrigerator until solid, then cut into 24 squares and enjoy.

Recipe provided with permission from the City of Nanaimo, which asked that it be noted, "From the people of Nanaimo to the world . . ."

Acknowledgements

This is my first book. It only came about because I had so much exceptional help and endless support from colleagues and friends and family.

My first round of thanks goes to the entire team at HarperCollins. Thank you, everyone, for helping me turn an idea into a book. I'm so very grateful. In particular, thanks to those who helped with iconic Canadian food: Noelle Zitzer, Lisa Rundle, Valerie Bailey, Leo MacDonald, Mike Mason, Inge "Operation Pork Buns" Siemens and Terry Toews. Jaline Tanne and Guy Dubois lent a hand, too: many thanks!

My editor, Brad Wilson, was the first to spot a book in me; thank you for your careful guidance and constant encouragement. To Judy Phillips, thank you for your gentle hand and meticulous edits; I couldn't have hoped for a better person to take the manuscript to the finish line.

Lots of thanks also to Alan Jones, whose hard work and expertise made the book look so smart and stylish. Noelle Zitzer and Kelly Hope, thank you for your creative eyes and attention to detail and for ensuring that everything was in its proper place.

Many, many thanks to Christopher Campbell; your beautiful photography is truly the other half of this book. Thanks, too, to Dennis Wood and Philip Buckley for all your skills and all the laughs in the photo studio. It was a joy to work with all three of you; that you are now friends is one of the best parts of writing this book.

I'm grateful for the support and encouragement of friends and editors at the *Toronto Star,* particularly Amy Pataki, whose witty responses about life as a restaurant critic added so much to the book; Rita Daly, who has been a mentor and friend from the beginning; and the tireless editors of the *Star*'s Life section, who work hard to give my column, "The Dish," such a great home.

I'm also endlessly grateful to Kim Honey, editor extraordinaire, who got me started down this road.

To my team of expert readers, Zannat Reza, Carol Harrison and Shannon Crocker, thank you: thank you for your insight, expertise and enthusiasm; it would have been impossible to finish this project without it and without you.

My wonderful friend Nora Hammond gets a big hug and thank you for reading the entire manuscript during a very busy time in her life.

I am so thankful for my family, who have been a constant in my life—not just for the last year of book writing but for always and everything. Thank you Mum, Dad, Caroline, Ryan and Lauren.

And finally my heartfelt and enduring thanks to Jeff, my best friend, whose unfailing faith in me is my greatest strength. Thank you for everything this past year.

Index